THE BRILLIANT FUNCTION OF PAIN

THE BRILLIANT FUNCTION OF PAIN

by

Milton Ward

"PAIN IS DESIGNED TO KEEP US *WELL*. . ."

A Yogic Understanding of Pain

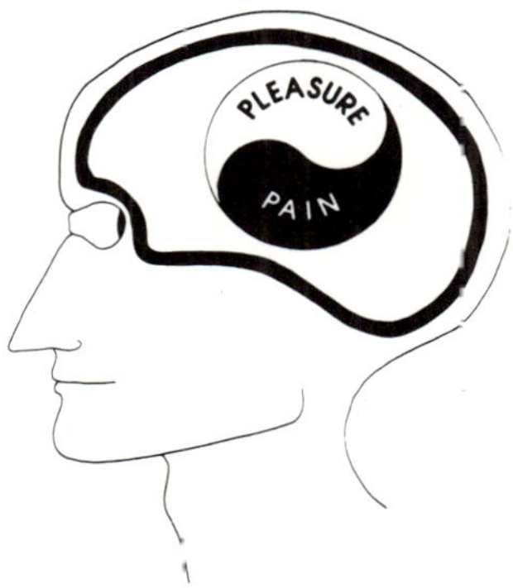

Published by

Optimus Books

Plaza Hotel, N.Y., N.Y.

&

CSA Press

Lakemont, Ga. 30552

Library of Congress Catalog Card Number 76-47432
Standard Book Number 0-87707-194-2

Printed for the Publisher by
CSA Printing & Bindery, Lakemont, Georgia 30551

To Dr. Ramamurti S. Mishra and to Swami Satchidananda, my teachers, and to all other spiritual physicists, past and present, whose sacrifice and legacy we are only beginning to comprehend.

CONTENTS

Introduction 9

Chapter One — The Terror of Pain. 11

Chapter Two — Guidance or Affliction 14

Chapter Three — What Is Pain?. 17

Chapter Four — The Subtle Intimations of Pain 20

Chapter Five — This Moment. 23

Chapter Six — Physical Problems 26

Chapter Seven — Emotional Imbalance 51

Chapter Eight — Mental Difficulty. 60

Chapter Nine — Spiritual Anguish. 63

Chapter Ten — Love and Sexual Frustration 73

Chapter Eleven — Artistic and Spontaneity Block 83

Chapter Twelve — Faith Healing, Tranquilizers, Bio-Feedback, Recreation. 87

Chapter Thirteen — The Malaise and the Rage of Modern Society. 90

Chapter Fourteen — Summary. .92

Chapter Fifteen — Conclusion 94

INTRODUCTION

How do most of us deal with pain? We either fight it or justify it. Many of us do both. But very few *make full use* of pain. Those who utilize its brilliant function are closer to their reality. They are intuitive, healthier, happier and more effective beings.

The people who fight pain run to an endless succession of doctors, therapists and religious healers. They demand any treatment that will promptly relieve them of their suffering. Many of these pain fighters also go to great extremes to *prevent* pain. They jog and meditate and add wheat germ to their cereal every morning. But all these pain fighters are running scared. Despite all their efforts, pain keeps catching up with them. It remains a persistent enemy. As much as they try, they can neither prevent nor defeat the aches, sickness, depressions and world malaise with which they are doing battle.

The justifiers *rationalize* pain. God is testing us, they proclaim, we must carry our cross. Like Job they *trust* God's intentions. Other mystically minded justifiers gaze down from their Himalayan heights and proclaim that pain and pleasure are identical. They tell us we can't have one without the other. All these justifiers enjoy tremendous highs when they are convinced their faith transcends this world. But they also suffer abysmal lows. The precise merit system by which God inflicts or withholds pain eludes them. And when they confront the suffering of the world, they are *doubly dejected*; in addition to their normal pains they must endure the black torment of disillusionment.

So that it would appear that for the vast majority of us, pain has no purpose and also no lasting antidote. Is this so? If we touch a burning stove, the purpose of pain is abundantly clear. Pain is a warning system, an internal guidance system. Unceasingly, every single moment, the pain-pleasure principle dictates our activity. We cannot eat one excess slice of bread or deprive ourselves of one hour of sleep without getting appropriate pain messages. Every action is accompanied by an equally strong reaction. We make all kinds of detours but our uncompromising reality greets us with the appropriate consequence in short order. The reaction or *karma* fits the detour precisely, the punishment fits the crime. We are governed by an overwhelming reality and its name is pain.

Our premise in this volume is that pain has *astounding logic* and *distinct function*. The great secret of the East is *awareness*. Awareness of *what is*: of feeling, of pain or release from pain; of the subtle reality that underlies our apparent reality. There is an overwhelming wisdom here that is more profound than all our scientific and spiritual cogitation. It encompasses and unifies our physical, emotional, mental and spiritual being.

Like so many of the books that stream from the hands of esoterics, this volume will occasionally presume on your credibility. The test of its truth is not cold assessment by the mind. It must be tested experientially, or it is not worth your time.

A word of urgent warning must conclude this introduction. Anyone who doesn't make full use of every possible professional help is a fool. But we are equal fools if we do not use the instinctive signals which rise from our inner feelings. What we must avoid are professional experts who deny the existence of our instincts, and esoteric extremists who deny the value of highly trained and experienced physicians, psychologists and theologians. To suggest that these two are mutually exclusive camps, or to insist that any single discipline is heir to all the secrets of the universe, is an absurd lie.

Chapter One

THE TERROR OF PAIN

We all suffer pain. Not a day goes by, hardly an hour, without some heart stabbing pain. Even if we are filled with a thousand joys, something will arise to shatter us. King or pauper, old or young, successful or a failure—a headache, a disappointment, a quarrel, the eyes of an aging loved one, the world situation—*something* will pierce the marrow of our being.

Because of this pain, many of us are a mess. We are physically, emotionally, mentally or spiritually wracked. All that sustains us is hope—hope that our latest doctor, psychologist, therapy, religious faith, diet or drug will lift us out of our pain. One thousand previous hopes have left us as miserable as ever but we move on to the avalanche of new remedies. New therapies, this year's crop of "how to" books, a pain killing drug, martial arts, a faith healer, a new social, business or artistic interest to distract us—there is always a new panacea. It may be just a suggestion from a corny Reader's Digest article, a bit of mysticism from a Tibetan monk, a chance remark, and once again we have *hope*!

Initially we are helped. The new discipline does some good. Our spirits are lifted. We give the new hope our undying faith. We try to convert every relative, every friend, every stranger to our great discovery. But then the tired phrases turn meaningless. The new disciplines become a burden or they have a bad side effect. Our great "truth" is no longer the answer. We need another *hope*.

No problem! The pain careerists, the healers, thousands of them are waiting for us with open arms. So all knowing, so superior, urging us to buy their *sure thing*. And somehow we *know*, or soon enough find out, that they too have no ultimate solutions; that piecemeal treatment of this or that individual difficulty is a patchwork action. It doesn't do the job.

Why? Because most remedies are *imposed*, intruded on our natural selves. They are manipulations that create three selves where previously there was one self. In accepting a remedy you become the you who *is*, plus the you who is helping you become *other* than the you who *is*, plus the you whom you hope to *become*. This multi-character often creates confusion which is far greater than your original difficulty. You are at constant odds with yourself. You also develop a terrible ambivalence towards the healer who is helping you. You want to give this expert your fervent support but you can't suppress feelings of hatred because he is interfering with your self-motivation.

Where does all this start? Can we avoid this proliferation of confusion? Is there an answer to pain? An honest, lasting answer? Or is the book you are reading right this minute another overlay of advice that will *add* to your burden?

Do I recommend organic foods, exercise, outdoor life, jogging, astrology, hormones, water therapy or any of a thousand other cure-alls? I most certainly do not! What good are organic foods or vitamins if you are not aware that the pain in your stomach is rejecting *any food*? What do we have to gain from exercise or outdoor living if we do not have enough awareness to open a pants belt that is constricting our breathing, blocking our food digestion and forcing our heart to double its work in order to pump blood through our impeded arteries? What purpose does my ability to play tennis serve if I disregard the pleadings of my body to quit endangering my heart muscles after four brutal sets of singles?

I have nothing to recommend to you, absolutely nothing except what you yourself are prepared to learn from the enormous wisdom of your incredible inner self. The strongest preventive force, the *one preventive mechanism* that never stops working for us is our instinct. All healers agree that this is so. When they recommend a vacation or some rest, they are encouraging us to function out of instinct. They are conceding that there are inner capacities that infinitely exceed all learned knowledge.

Why do we fail to use these capacities? The main culprit is our misunderstanding of pain, our failure to respond to its message. When we suffer pain, we immediately and automatically label it *sickness*. Actually, it is a *brilliant signal*. It is "telling" us to do something to *right ourselves*. And, as we shall learn, it is "telling" us *what* to do—minute by minute—with amazing accuracy—to prevent the more serious problems that will require radical outside help.

Pain is not a terror. Quite the opposite. It reminds us that an infinitely brilliant force, *our own force*, is functioning in our behalf. It is, when we begin to perceive it, a wonderful reminder of a vast spectrum of consciousness that lies beyond the limited perception of our thought process.

Chapter Two

GUIDANCE OR AFFLICTION?

Is there an uncomplicated way to gain health, to be effective in your work, in your social relationships, in your hobbies? Can you achieve a high state of perception, a sustained feeling of purpose and pleasure in this puzzling world? Can this be done without creating more serious complications than the difficulties you are trying to discharge? Yes we can, but we have allowed ourselves to be deceived. We have discarded our innate physical, mental and spiritual wisdom. In this world of specialization, we hand all our symptoms to experts, without stopping to ask ourselves if this is always the best course.

The key to this disaster is our reaction to pain. We regard pain as a bitter enemy. Not so! If we wouldn't freeze at the very thought of pain, we would find it to be a wonderful friend, designed to *assist us*, not to give us grief. *We must regain our capacity to perceive the logic of pain, to trust our pain.* I believe there may have been a time, many years ago, when mankind reacted to pain as automatically as forest animals or birds do today, with simple reflex mechanism. I believe it was a time of utmost wisdom.

Our greatest mistake is our inability to see that pain is a guide, not an affliction. Pain points to the condition or ailment, *it is not the ailment*. This is true of all pain: body, mind, emotion or spirit. Actually pain is a good sign. It is an indication that our being is *correcting itself*. Pain is a warning system. It is also an efficient *guiding system*. More often than not, the cure for the problem *is indicated by the pain*. We search everywhere for cures and our brilliant inner nature is pointing to specific action.

Am I saying that all experts should be disregarded? Not at all! But we should be more inclined to those specialists who do not rob us of our own awareness mechanism. You may ask, "But how can I avoid seeking help when I have a serious disease or an organic injury?" You can't. Such matters require handling by highly trained people. But you *will find* that your failure to "read" earlier pain guides may have led to the more complex problem you have today.

"But how can I rely on myself to "read" these lesser pain alarms?" you ask. To a degree we do this all the time. If we feel severe chills or fatigue, we go to bed to head off illness. A more acute capacity to respond to these pain signals is the object of this book.

Still you ask, "What difference will it make if I improve my response to pain signals? Isn't it safer to share my problems with experts *before* these problems become severe?" Yes and no. Reliance on experts becomes a habit. When we constantly hand this responsibility away, we no longer bother to *analyze our pains*.

Pain awareness is hardly new. It is as old as man. But it is becoming increasingly popular in the West. We are rejecting the robot life style which consumerism promotes. Various psychological techniques, Yoga and other self analysis disciplines have fueled this revolt. Millions of people are discovering that the book knowledge and advice of our medical and spiritual pundits is often no match for a high level of intuitive and experiential awareness.

These people are saying, "The inner being *tells us*, we do not tell it." They are reminding us that any apparatus which is composed of about one hundred trillion parts (human cells) in several thousand varieties, which performs a fantastic number of electronic, chemical and atomic functions, which beats our hearts and expands our lungs, which digests our food, which sees, hears and thinks, which can create a complete new human being—*knows very well* what it is doing.

I do not intend to make this book a debate between natural healers and the acknowledged medical and spiritual advice givers. It *is* my intention to help you *prove to yourself* whether or not your pain signals do in fact guide you to a more resilient and happy existence. You can only do this experientially. You *cannot* do this theoretically. In the chapters that follow, I will ask you to search out your most subtle pains to determine what they ask of you. I may suggest possibilities but the answers *must come from you*.

I am not suggesting that you become your own doctor or psychiatrist or minister. I am suggesting that your feelings, your pains and your instincts can make their job much easier. I insist that your health, your well being, your outlook can be improved several times over if you simply "listen" to your amazing self.

Chapter Three

WHAT IS PAIN?

Search the medical and psychological literature for a definition of pain. You will find a great deal of equivocation. You will read, on the one hand, that pain is largely subjective because it varies with the individual. You will find that the word *psychosomatic* serves as a convenient catch-all, though the word does little to explain pain. It merely suggests that there is a mysterious place in the psyche that somehow affects the physical body. You will read that organic pain, such as bodily injury or a burn, is understood to result from nerve ending injury. But there is candid and virtually unanimous agreement that all these are only sketchy definitions of pain. Western science admits that it is at a loss to explain precisely what it is when a person registers pain.

Freud wrote in a volume titled, *Beyond the Pleasure Principle*: (1920) London: Hogarth Press, 1948.

> We would readily express our gratitude to any philosophical or psychological theory which was able to inform us of the meaning of the feelings of pleasure and unpleasure which act so imperatively upon us.

Another psychiatrist, Thomas S. Szasz, who made a considerable study of pain, writes in his book, *Pain and Pleasure* (1957, 1975 New York: Basic Books, Inc.

> . . . our modern society tends to misinterpret pain by presuming that everyone who complains of pain is "sick" either mentally or physically.

In the same book he writes:

> A simple back pain is treated differently by the family physician (who might use drugs), by a neurosurgeon, by a chiropractor, by a psychiatrist, by a masseur and by a faith healer.

What we have is confusion. Our contemporary society, which is so desperately concerned with the alleviation of pain, has no idea *what pain is*, and cannot understand why pain responds to techniques that seem so opposite to one another. Reluctantly we concede that a multitude of factors may be involved in pain such as a patient's subjective mind, muscle tone, nerve tone, bone structure, blood stream, education, faith, etc. But we have been too busy seeking and marketing cures to take the time to define the enemy. Is it malingering? Is it hypochondria? Is it an inexplicable mystery?

The East has a precise definition of pain which might be stated as follows:

> *Our instinctive being constantly emanates from and seeks a state of mental, emotional, physical and spiritual equilibrium. All pain is a request or demand to us (our minds) to help restore this equilibrium. It is a positive process.*

This definition declares that we have an instinctive self that will persist in subjecting us to pain if we do not bend to its needs, and will discontinue the pain if we adjust to its needs. Another corollary follows automatically—that unless we exist in the desired state of equilibrium, there will inevitably be pain. Further that pain is not an odd quirk of nature—meaningless, specious. Instead that nature uses pain as brilliantly and absolutely as it uses the laws of chemistry or physics; with infallible purpose.

Among the oriental non-dualists, both happiness and suffering are considered to be non-existent, in the sense that these are continuing, universal adjustments—ecological process. Pain is not a dormant condition. On the face of it, all this may appear to be beyond rational sanity. Do not judge this too quickly. Wait until you have experienced *your own* instinctive pain process.

Chapter Four

THE SUBTLE INTIMATIONS OF PAIN

Pain from a corn on our little toe tells us to change our shoes. The message is clear enough. It is *not* telling us we have inferior feet that are prone to corns. It is simply telling us to relieve the pressure of our shoe.

Can we perceive equally precise messages from our more subtle pains? For example, can we foretell the advent of a cold by catching the subtle discomforts that tell us to retreat from an obsessive work load, to get back to our center, to break off a masochistic attachment, to return to a strict diet of wholesome foods?

Is it possible that these measures will rebuild our resistance before the virus has a chance to gain an upper hand? I believe so. In my own case and in the case of others who develop this symptom sensitivity, the incidence of colds is substantially reduced or eliminated entirely. Is this lack of awareness the factor that makes certain people more cold prone than others?

This awareness succeeds in other areas. I have seen people give up cigarettes, drugs, liquor or excessive sweets after a few days of this pain awareness. Not by determination. Not by grit. But by allowing themselves to be acutely aware of their pain signals. Certainly the coughing, the dryness, the eye tearing, the aftertaste of cigarette smoking, all shout their unmistakable message. The taste of sweets, if one is truly aware, is actually bitter to the mouth. Liquor scalds the throat and gullet.

Subtle pains such as aches, depressions, performance jitters, shyness are also precise signal systems. They are not afflictions or malfunctions. They are not misfortunes. Does the pain of being shy make us a shy person? Or is each uncomfortable feeling demanding that we be our *natural self*? Do performance jitters declare that we are chronic nervous nellies or are they repeating over and over again, "Trust your moment, trust your moment, take your rightful place!"

Is the pain of excessive worry a sign that we are uncontrolled worriers, or is it crying out to us to quit laying indecision on our heads and to go along with whatever comes along? If we hit a tennis ball badly, is the sharp feeling of inadequacy telling us we are choked-up players, or is it simply saying, "You are playing without any respect for your game. Why? Stop crowding the ball." Is sleeplessness telling us we are hopeless insomniacs? Or is our edginess telling us we require solid rest? All of us know the feeling of instant sleep, as much as ten times a day, when we are on a restful vacation. These and other examples are discussed at length in later chapters.

There are more subtle signals. For example, the feeling of being "turned on," of being "in our vibe" is known to all of us. It is a sense of clarity, of effortlessly riding on a subtle hum, of being at peace with the world. This is the constant aim of our brilliant being. The Yogis describe it as a spiritual state, "existing in *nadam*." Scientists use the word homeostasis. Whether it is material or spiritual, nobody denies that we are dealing with a *reality*. How do we harness this brilliant entity or force? Is it possible that the laws that govern our psyche are as brilliant, as quick, as absolute as the laws that govern the atom or the action of light?

As we study this process, (what the Easterners call the *tantric* function) the incessant return to equilibrium in all things including our being, we feel a growing excitement over the sanity of our inner world. It has an exalting effect on our entire outlook.

But it isn't easy. We are not discussing a quick preventive or remedial action. We are describing a positive response day after day, year after year. We are *all* blessed with this automatic response. But those who spontaneously utilize pain to *utmost advantage*, are the most successful people among us, the best athletes, the top performers, the easygoing business people, the most admired public figures. Pain never throws them. It is a constant aid.

Can pain avoid more serious disease: pneumonia, heart attack, cancer, psychosis? Long term constriction of our systems by prolonged physical and emotional tension undermines our resistance. Is it possible that early response to this constriction could have avoided the disease? Does our brilliant being transmit intimations that anticipate these ailments before they become serious?

The medical community has tested thousands of drugs, medical devices, surgical treatments. Have they tested a holistic response to pain? Have they investigated the benefits of feeling-guided equilibrium?

Our minds cannot begin to cope with the infinite complexities of existence. A high level of feeling awareness, including pain, provides infinitely more intelligent response than our one-thought-after-another-thought linear mind. Those of us who observe people with acute feeling response—those of us who cultivate this awareness—find conclusive evidence of disease resistant capacity.

Chapter Five

THIS MOMENT

Positive response to pain must be experienced if it is to be understood. As an exercise let us experience *this moment*. You are reading this book. You are not conscious of any pain, so you think. But if you examine yourself, you may discover a number of pains. Perhaps you must go to the bathroom. Your bladder or your lower bowel is sending this message to you by transmitting a form of pain. Many of us neglect even this fundamental pain for hours, causing damage to the nervous system, the urinary tract and the intestinal tract. Is some article of clothing pressuring your body? Perhaps you want to pull off your shoes or your tie. Now, as you scan your body further, do you find any area of tension? Is your hand or back contorted? Are you being asked to adjust your body position, to place a pillow behind your head?

It may be that the tension in your hand or back has nothing to do with your body position. Take this moment to examine the pain which you feel. If you concentrate on this pain, you may discover that it relates to a personal conflict. If you concentrate on the pain (not the pros and cons of the conflict) for several additional moments, you may be surprised. The pain will actually point to a very logical handling of the conflict itself. (Please do not accept or reject this notion until you test it. And remember to concentrate on the pain, not the situation.)

Perhaps you now feel an obscure, shadowy pain. You find that you are very impatient at this moment. Your impatience is an emotional difficulty. Put the book down. *Do not* enter into a big debate with yourself on the cause of your impatience. But *do* concentrate on the pain that it causes. Again, you may be surprised. The pain that is caused by your impatience will actually reveal a precise resolution for your impatience problem. The chances are good that you will discover that you have no personal conflict and that you have no impatience problem at all. These were labels which you attached to *the very pain that was trying to rid you of these notions.*

You may feel now that there is an amazing stabilizing force within yourself. You feel good, too good in fact. It worries you. You think you have *no right* to feel so good. You tell yourself it is temporary. You test this concept on other physical, mental or emotional problems. Again you concentrate on the pain, not the thoughts you have regarding the pain, and again it works.

Now you decide that you *can't possibly* be problem free. *Nobody* is problem free! Our world is a *constant* problem! It is filled with disappointment: war, poverty, atom bombs, racism, sickness and death. "What," you ask, "can this inner stabilizing force do about our spiritual bankruptcy?" For many years you have been trying to find a satisfactory explanation for nature's game or God's purpose. You haven't found a solid explanation. Like all of us, you feel occasional futility. What can concentration on the pain of futility provide?

Try it! Take your attention away from all the debates between atheists and religionists, between one religion and another religion, between your love for this world and your disillusion. Instead concentrate on your black pain, your *Weltschmerzen* (world pain). Feel it in your heart ache. Feel it in your gut. Again you may be surprised. Perhaps, like the Hindus and Buddhists you will sense that there is neither pain nor pleasure. Or that there is a long and a short view of our existence. Perhaps you will sense nothing that can be put into words; an unmanifest world within the manifest world. For this moment your instinctive self will somehow guide you to becoming one *with* the world—instead of being one *against* the world.

Perhaps you sense now that our object is not to deal with pain but rather to let pain deal with us. You sense that our pain actually *commands* us to live vibrant, fulfilled, outgoing, *painless* lives.

Chapter Six

PHYSICAL PROBLEMS

How do we avoid and overcome physical problems? To what degree do our pain signals help this process? What precise techniques should we utilize to take full advantage of these signals?

We imagine we suffer breakdowns in our health from some single cause. Actually, most ailments come from a systemic breakdown which is caused by a *combination of factors*. Individually these items may seem insignificant; lack of sleep, a dull outlook, overwork, stuffing our stomachs, lack of exercise, allowing ourselves to be overheated, unresolved tensions. All these may appear to be temporary difficulties that can readily be overcome. It is not that easy. Unless we deal with these matters promptly, we are caught in a downslide. When these conditions combine and act on each other, we find ourselves *severely* depleted, candidates for *major* physical problems.

It is one of the main premises of this book that our pain signals help us to avoid cumulative illness. But there are *so many* discomfort signals. Muscle aches, nerve pain, skin pain, sweating, headache, nausea, stuffed feeling, cramps, chills, overheating, coughing, itching, tiredness, loginess, breathlessness—on and on it goes. Must we react to each and every one of these pangs? Wouldn't we become hypochondriacs?

Not if our pain response is instinctive. Dogs and cats, at least until they are spoiled by humans, eat one modest meal a day. They do not *tell themselves* that such a diet will keep them slim or sexually attractive. They do it *without thinking*. When they are even slightly ill, they refuse *all food*. Are they smarter than us despite our more highly developed brains? How do they manage their self control? *Instinctively* their stomach *tells them* it is satisfied. Instinctively they prefer a light, unstuffed feeling to the pleasure that food might give to their tongue or ego.

We suffer the tortures of the damned after a too heavy meal. For hours, if not days, our body screams at us never to do this again. Yet we go on doing it. Are we unaware of our body's rejection of the food? Not at all! If we examine our feelings as we gulp excess food, *we do* sense clear indication of nausea and repulsion. The message is there *before* we eat, *as* we eat and *after* we eat. But *still* we gorge ourselves.

Too much heat or clothing on our body tells us to adjust our clothing or to adjust the thermostat. Exercising to excess or exercise that strains particular muscles causes immediate pain signals. We receive a variety of signals that are precise and constant, whether or not we regard them.

The body also insists on being *used*. It rejects un-use as precisely as it rejects abuse. Palpitation, itchiness, lack of energy, lack of suppleness are all clear-cut demands for use. Our body is saying, "Get some exercise. Cut the lawn. Use these muscles. Use this body." Most of us respond. Yet millions of people believe that the queasy feeling of un-use indicates that they are soft, lazy, physically weak. They are mistaking the symptom for the problem. Their response to pain is distorted.

There is a reverse side to this coin. There are very clear signs of *physical ease*. If we feel exhilarated, a glowing well-being, a free flowing vibe from head to toe, a body suppleness, an unencumbered bowel, a sweet, clean feeling in our mouth, a fresh sensation in the back of our nose that tingles down the spine with each breath, clear eyes, clear headedness—we have physical ease as opposed to physical dis-ease. Anything less is a demand from our brilliant body for some action on our part. "Unless you are feeling that equilibrium," it is saying, "you are not heeding your instinct." Once you regain your equilibrium, you will be devoid of *all your hypochondria.* You will be in a state of expanded consciousness in which your needs will be anticipated before you are greeted with more acute pain signals and you will respond automatically without thinking.

The point here is that prevention and cure require a holistic approach for which pain and lack of pain are the primary guides. The following pages list only a few among hundreds of physical problems. These examples indicate methods of approach rather than solutions. There are thousands of recommended cures. What good are all these cures if our basic approach is lacking?

The Common Cold

How often has your common cold been a blessing? Yes, even the misery of an endlessly running nose, of uncontrolled sneezing, of fiendish coughing, of four or five days of absolute *blah*—all turn out to be a bonus. You find yourself cleansed, surprisingly clear headed, physically attuned. You gain a new perspective towards your work, towards your family. You gain a sane perspective of *yourself.* And you have devoured a good book in the bargain.

The common cold makes you feel *totally vulnerable.* During its worst hours you wonder if you will actually survive. At a certain point it forces you to give up the fight. Total surrender! Nature is the *boss*! You are down to point zero, a very healthy place to be. This return to nothingness, our absolute surrender to instinct, may be the whole point of this remarkable exercise. The Vedics of India believe that zero is the state of highest wisdom. Devoid of all commitments, all compulsions, all tendencies—the horizon takes on a new look. All options are open and we are closest to the brilliance of that inner being which far outstrips the brilliance of our minds. We are somehow drained of cynicism. We are left with a new respect for our life, for *life*. Isn't it amazing that nature makes this corrective action with such bulls eye precision?

Could we have avoided this cold in the first place? I believe the answer is "Yes, if we had accomplished precisely what the cold accomplished." There are lucky people who almost never suffer from colds or flu. Are they blessed with the capacity to respond more immediately to their pain signals? Do they function more directly from their instinct; do they read their autonomic system more readily; are they closer to intuitive mind?

There are a large number of psychological, physical and emotional warnings of lowered resistance far in advance of a cold. This is hardly news to you, I am sure. But we disregard these alarm bells with hardly a thought. A lackluster feeling, *a one bell alarm*. Awareness of an emotional hang-up, *two bells*. A sense of compulsiveness, *three bells*. Disregard for our feelings, *four bells*. Weariness, sleeplessness, *five bells*. Headache, *six bells*. Chills, *seven bells*. An occasional sneeze, *eight bells*. Leaky nose, *nine bells*. The works, *ten bells*! Nature demands its full adjustment. The virus performs nature's job most efficiently.

During the pre-cold process, most of us hardly bother to respond. We feel our muscle system, nerve system, life force system constricting. We order a cup of tea with lemon instead of our usual coffee. We swallow a useless antihistamine. We don't bother to respond to something as fundamental as a bad case of chills. These chills are pleading with us to *stay warm*. But we wear skimpy or ersatz clothing, sleep under ersatz blankets, on ersatz mattresses, and watch our bodies constrict as if we have been issued a torture sentence by a kangaroo court. In fifty backward countries, "uneducated peasants" respond to cold discomfort by wearing heavy shoes, wool socks, wool underwear and clothing, some animal outer garment. They sleep under and over genuine covering, not phony thermal blankets or cotton mattresses. We have advanced beyond these poor souls.

To completely slow down, to cleanse the stomach and body of excess food waste, to sleep a day or two, to get genuinely comfortable, to quit playing the tension game, to allow constricted lungs, muscles, nerves, arteries, life force to work freely is somehow anti-heroic in our society. Sickness is a heroism—flirting with fate—using our pain to prove our martyrdom instead of using it for its intended purpose.

Long Term Orthopedic Pain

Muscle, nerve, tendon and other orthopedic pain is a universal complaint. Half the population appears to be suffering from some form of backache or sciatica. Mineral baths, saunas, masseurs, chiropractors, osteopaths, orthopedists, physical therapists and psychologists hold out their special promise. But millions of people silently bear this harrowing misery.

Instinct awareness, or pain awareness, can be remarkably helpful. One may experience the pain in both an immobile and an active state. For our purpose let us hypothetically respond to a backache that causes sciatic nerve pain in the leg as well.

If you are afflicted with such a pain and are sitting in a comfortable chair or lying on a bed, the usual tendency is to change to a position that appears to be less painful, or to flex the aching area, or perhaps take a pill, or ultimately to seek outside help. Suppose we try something entirely different. We are going to focus our concentration so as to experience *every possible pain tremor*. This is more easily said than done. We tend to lose this concentration very quickly. We twist away from the pain by making some nervous movement. Or some thought distracts us. In order to be successful we must *hold this concentration*.

If you have any long-term painful area, you may wish to try this right now. Hold your utmost concentration on the very core of the pain. Go deeper and deeper into the pain. Then, with ample patience respond to the intent of the pain (not your mind intent) as precisely as you possibly can. (I am not suggesting that you flex the muscles around the pain for some temporary relief. We do this all the time and it doesn't help at all.) If you do this correctly the response will be far more subtle and far more meaningful. Give yourself four or five minutes to become the absolute servant of the pain.

I would guess, at the very least, that you have gained an altogether new familiarity and insight into your pain. Perhaps you achieved much more. You may have found yourself making a very profound adjustment in a mysteriously internal way. Did you feel a strange regrouping of some muscle or nerve system? Was it hardly perceptible yet remarkably right? Did you appear to return to some *essential* self? Is it astonishing that you may have subjected this condition to every possible therapy except the therapy which the pain itself was seeking?

Years of living with a bad back will not be overcome with one such awareness experience. It may take a few weeks but you will find it remarkably effective. This should be coupled with awareness concentration while you are actively *using* the limb that aches. If it is a back problem, you may know that extended walking or even standing in one place for more than a short time causes fierce binding, stabbing pains and numbness. Now let us try an extended walk with maximum pain concentration.

The key here is *not to wait*, as we normally do, for the pain to become severe before we allow it to rise to our consciousness. Instead we will watch for the very first scintilla of pain. And we will respond to this pain signal *no matter how slight it is*. The pain may ask you to slow down in your walking very considerably. It may demand that you release your abdomen. It may suggest a quite unexpected change in your leg or foot motion, or indicate that the physical problem is entirely related to a job situation or a personal anxiety. Or a thousand other possibilities.

Once again it is the internal request of the pain, subtle

as it is, that we must satisfy. Not some chance suggestion that comes to the mind. The pain signal "knows absolutely" what it wants. If it receives our full concentration, there will be improvement. We may find ourselves walking twice the usual distance without severe pain.

This awareness may have more to tell us. Perhaps the muscle-nerve system in the limb has been inhibited for several years. The pain persists. The return to normal use may not be that easy. We must now fulfill further requests.

Our pain may be demanding that we move even deeper to the core of the pain, to ask it where it is available for release, where it is ready to replace its binding tendency with full function. And finally, even this may be insufficient. The ultimate request may be for a return to enthusiasm, unqualified pleasure in every movement, an end to *all restrictions.*

How often muscle and nerve pain disappear when we lose ourselves in a game of tennis, fully let go on the dance floor, are enthralled by a happy vacation; when we love ourselves, love others and love our world. Ultimately our pain calls on us to charge into pleasurable, spontaneous, totally unselfconscious movement, born in the timeless grace of our original self; to skip, to run, to swing our arms, to become interpretive dancers with unqualified freedom is the ultimate injunction of physical pain, to climb that forest path with delight, to swing that racket with devastating abandon, to be in that mysterious zone where the body does it, not we!

We may lack sufficient oils in the body, we may have a vitamin deficiency, we may benefit from massage, acupuncture, osteopathic or chiropractic or orthopedic treatment, we may be helped by zitz baths and a hundred other remedies. But what good are all these, if we are not bowled over by the fact and mystery and mad joy of our life and all life?

From a preventive standpoint, a great deal of misery could be avoided if we would pause briefly, whenever we are engaged in physical effort, to receive the instructions of our inner system. We can learn immediately whether we are creating trouble for ourselves. Any physical activity that is pursued with obstinate disregard of pain or emotional tension will wreak havoc. The activity will be accomplished with infinitely less effort if our muscle, tendon and nerve systems are motivated by that inner sanity with which we are all blessed.

The Strains of Exercise and Sports

If there is pain in exercise, the pain is telling us *not* to proceed. Or we are being asked to attempt the same exercise without pain. This will be challenged by many who will say that unless we feel pain, we will never extend our capacities and endurance. They will insist that any contrary statement is a cop-out.

They are dead wrong. Most exercise is done to excess in our society. Sports, calisthenics, jogging, often do much harm. Even yoga students stretch their tendons to a point beyond sound judgment. All this is unnecessary. *Any goal in sports or exercise can be achieved without strain more easily than it can be achieved with strain.*

Most of us suffer calisthenics as an unpleasant duty, largely because we make it a painful effort. We can't imagine painless calisthenics. We prefer competitive sports in which the excitement covers over the pain. But we come off the playing courts with muscle and tendon pains that last for days and cause lifetime injury. Is there such a thing as painless exercise that *builds* the body and *develops proficiency* in a sport at the same time? Yes there is.

The method is quite simple. *We heed the pain!* Take any exercise that you do regularly: calisthenics, golf, tennis, even weight lifting. Intensify your awareness. If you feel any pain, even the slightest excess body tension, allow the pain to alter the exercise slightly so that the pain is eliminated. In most cases, this will not occur unless there is a certain spontaneity in the action, a slight sense of improvisation. Whatever is done with mental exertion is also done with pain.

If you constantly adjust the exercise to *release* you from the pain, you will experience a rush of energy throughout your body, a continuous "physical high." You will be astonished at the ease and proficiency with which you execute complex maneuvers which previously caused such trouble. "But," you may ask, "is this the way to achieve form? Form *cannot* be improvised." This is correct. The acquiring of good form takes great effort. But unless we ultimately execute this form with ease, unless the body and mind make the effort with a certain pleasure—an innate élan—we perform poorly. Neither form nor spontaneity can do without the other.

There is also a mental-emotional factor in sports which turns so many players into losers rather than winners. We all hit bad shots. We all fall behind in a game. This causes frustration, impatience, dejection . . . pain. Some people contend with this pain, others choke up and blow the game. This is largely due to incorrect interpretation of their pain. A badly hit ball causes self-assessment. This self-assessment should say, "You're crowding the ball. You should have stepped back and taken an easier swing." *So that the discomfort actually points to the mistake and offers a solution to the mistake*. This discomfort will emanate from the exact portion of the body that performed awkwardly.

Poor players read an entirely different message into the pain, a kind of screaming self-condemnation. "You're falling apart. You're a suffering person and a losing person!" They have totally twisted its meaning. It doesn't take long for them to proceed to, "You're a hopeless dolt, an inferior player and an inferior person." Is it any wonder they choke up? Natural endowment, talent, inclination and training are vital to ability in sports. But those who make positive use of their pain signals are superior performers.

Any discussion of exercise must include mention of yoga *asanas* or *hatha* yoga, as it is called. This remarkable practice has added a new dimension to our concept of exercise. *Hatha* yoga is designed to stretch and limber the body, to massage the internal organs and to strengthen the muscle system. But its primary function is to bring us to an acute state of *body* and *breath awareness*. It is a physical meditation. A position is taken and held. While it is being held, we are able to probe for pain spots and to gradually respond to this pain. Hatha yoga could be called a pain scanner. Any stiffness is immediately revealed and gradually overcome.

Those who suffer long term body pains should not be scared away from yoga exercises. A backache, for example, forces us to immobilize other parts of the body. If this goes on for any length of time, these other body parts are weakened. In the end, this may more severely strain the backache. Imagine a hammock with one torn cord. If all the other cords are strong, the hammock will continue to support our body. But several worn cords will throw the hammock out of shape and impose an even greater strain on the bad cord. Hatha yoga permits us to keep all parts of the body strong. Ultimately, this greatly benefits the originally afflicted part.

Headache

Headache is said to be the most common physical ailment there is. I doubt if the devil himself could invent any lingering pain comparable to the hellish, gnawing, debilitating torment of a headache. It is estimated that a majority of our population have painful headaches at least once a week.

I firmly believe that we can eliminate our headaches with ease. Most headache is a supplemental warning system. If we do not respond to warning signals from our stomach, to the torture of compulsiveness, to the overexcitement of emotionalism, to the strain of overwork, our nature utilizes the pain of a headache to provide a second jolt to slow us down.

Headache is a response to constriction—any and all kinds of constriction. It is as if the brain can take just so much constriction elsewhere before it constricts *itself*. Among those who practice the various forms of physical and meditational yoga, headache is almost non-existent. There is nothing mysterious or occult in this. These people have a more acute awareness of their pain symptoms. And they respond to these symptoms before constriction extends to the head. They can more readily sense inner resistance to an excess of food or liquor, to compulsiveness, to over-excitement, and give in to this resistance *promptly*. This belief in the *self* is virtually the sum total of all the mysterious objectives and benefits of Eastern theory.

But suppose you *already have* the headache, that you feel terrible. All feeling of equilibrium has evaporated. You have *lost* your wonderful internal sense—that sense which makes all existence meaningful, logical, humorous, intangibly yet most tangibly okay. Did this loss cause the headache, or did the headache cause this loss? The former, of course.

By now this contraction of your life force is feeding on itself. Perhaps it has been going on for some time. Your life style has become compulsive. Your habits have been born of distaste and self hate. Does all this bad feeling, this closed heart, this being a slave to your senses, represent an unavoidable breakdown? Or is it demanding a realignment, a return to *nadam*, the OM vibration, that highly subtle, intuitive "I" current that presides over our being when we are on top of the world, a sense of our all-encompassing reality, a supra-mundane state.

Are most headaches due to a tightening of our channels, a blocking of current that will not be denied, an overheated circuit? Is this current so dictatorial that it utilizes the pain and misery of the headache to force us into some dark place to un-constrict ourselves? Is a migraine headache the *only effective medicine*—the only adequate dosage for extreme compulsiveness?

Most of us automatically reach for an aspirin. But

drugs only temporarily block the constriction. An inner frailty continues to slow us down. Ultimately we suffer the exact amount of reduced function (reduced eating, reduced overwork, etc.) we require. Every minute we are laid low is in effect a minute of restoration.

The punishment for violations to our instinct is not *for* the sins committed but *by* the sins committed. With simple experimentation and self-analysis, with respect for our pain signals wherever they appear initially, we can all achieve a headache free existence. The means by which we can develop acute sensitivity to any sign of constriction in other parts of the body psyche are covered in later chapters of this book.

Overeating and Harmful Foods

Millions of us find it impossible to keep our weight down. Almost *all of us* can't stop eating harmful foods. I would guess that three quarters of our population are uncontrolled food or liquor freaks.

Ultimately our eating can only be dictated by *ourselves*. Others may offer suggestions but only *you* and *I* can determine our food intake. Diet fads and outside advice are useless if they cause us to relinquish our *self-guidance*. How often do we eat badly because we are not in touch with our needs; or even as an act of spite because we were denied an instinctive response to food in childhood and finally relinquished this right entirely?

It is almost impossible to avoid all the food temptation around us. It takes Herculean effort to resist the advertising pressure by food manufacturers, and the host or hostess who would consider our refusal of food a lack of social courtesy. So we eat blindly. Our body may *demand* that we quit eating or change our diet. Our tongue and mouth may be anything but sweet tasting; our stomach may be anything but sweet feeling. We are suffering terrible digestive discomfort—stuffiness, heartburn, lack of appetite, lack of energy from lack of proper nourishment, loss of taste-feeling, coated tongue. But still we eat atrociously.

The rewards of sensible, truly instinctive eating are a far healthier body, a more alert mind, a calm emotional outlook, a more ample sexuality, and a more sensitive spiritual vibration. We all know that this top-of-the-world buoyancy is one hundred times more rewarding than an epicurean feast. But most of us can't get a handle on some means of permanent self-guidance and become idiot slaves to food.

How *do we* overcome this absurdity? The process isn't nearly as difficult as we are led to imagine. Wrestling with twenty different diets, feeling acute guilt when we eat a hundred extra calories, playing the food masochism game is infinitely more debilitating than instinctive response to food. Initially there should be a day or two of fasting on fruit juices to rest the stomach and restore the jaded palate. After that there are four simple rules:

1. Replace denuded food such as white flour products with food that is nourishing. Many people eat mountains of food because their body is searching for nourishment it might get from one bowl of rice or whole grains.

2. Examine your discomfort feelings. Any stomach pain, stuffiness, nausea is signalling you not to eat.

3. Pause briefly before each mouthful of food to ask yourself whether your stomach actually wants it. If you are merely satisfying your ego or palate, you will find that your stomach will reject the food.

4. Be aware of the taste of the food. If the taste of the food is abhorrent, do not swallow it.

Simple? Millions of people would have much happier, healthier, lives if they followed these four instinctive rules. And the hungry people of the world could be fed by the mountains of food we *shouldn't* eat. But we prefer to be depressed and diseased by the effects of overweight and stomach slop.

Your sense of smell and your taste buds also turn down *particular foods*. As you begin to perceive signals of rejection, you are amazed to find that foods you imagined to be your favorites are actually acrid tasting or bland. A discerning palate finds a bitter, repellent taste in anything made with sugar. It stings the tongue and throat. A highly developed palate can taste the presence of even a small amount of chemical product in a food. The mouth wishes to spit it out. Try eating a piece of cheap ersatz candy with concentration.

By pausing before we take anything into our mouth—by *thinking* about the taste, we are able to choose foods that *precisely* meet our needs at a particular time. This may appear to be stretching the point but experimentation will surprise you. Our body has amazing capacity to enormously desire food it needs and to reject food it does not want. The body requires food. If it can't get what it wants, it will take what it can get. But a food that it needs will send delicious feeling waves through our body. Under the right circumstances, an unjaded palate will find a fresh pear much better tasting than a *cordon bleu* soufflé. The body says quite clearly that it needs the life force in the pear and would be less happy with the hyped-up souffle.

Our instinct constantly chooses different foods under different circumstances. We instinctively vary our diet when there is colder or warmer weather, when we are unwell, when we are active or inactive, prior to a public appearance, and so on.

This same capacity can be employed to an even greater degree. Take a moment to imagine a particular food in your system. Gaze at it. Does it fill a clear need? Is there a vibratory indication that the food will affect you positively? There are an increasing number of body healers who ask us to hold a food or chemical in our hand and then measure muscle and other responses. I have observed immediate changes in body contraction resulting from the mere handling of a particular food or chemical. The electrochemical effect is surprising to observe, but should not startle us. We are each an amazing organism.

Is it farfetched to believe that our incredible cell system which can employ a single tiny atom to its purpose, should have the selective capacity to choose foods which enhance our body tone? For example, the Far Easterners have made a study of what they call *Yin* and *Yang* forces. For several hundreds of years, they have studied these balancing elements in nature. They maintain that this can also be experienced in our food intake. A diet composed of milk products, sugars, citrus fruits, white flower products and processed foods will make us excitable, overly vulnerable. They insist it will be accompanied by a less stable sexuality. They suggest that these foods should be balanced by *Yang* foods such as whole grains, bean products, meat, fish, when we want to restore animal stability to our being. This may hardly impress you at a first hearing, yet experimentation will surprise you. Or will it? Do we not instinctively *know* this to be true? Do we not tend to lighter *Yin* foods in the summer, and to *Yang* foods in the winter? Doesn't an athlete or a laborer prefer *Yang* foods? Don't we all feel the need to balance these *Yin* and *Yang* foods? Isn't this the precise instinctive process—the reaction to feeling, to comfort and discomfort which we are discussing? If we are able to do this, how much more precise can we become in this instinctive selective process?

Overweight and the eating of harmful foods will cease if we become acutely conscious of the wishes of our internal being. Ultimately our demand for a calm, light feeling in the stomach, for sound sleep uninterrupted by digestive storms, for a feeling of delight rather than remorse in our eating habits, for a quickness of being, are infinitely more persuasive than the short lived taste thrill which unneeded food provides.

Accommodating Infirmities

There are a large number of ailments that linger on for years. Though they leave us debilitated and may ultimately seriously undermine our health, they pose no immediate danger to our lives. Included among these are such sicknesses as arthritis, sinusitis, allergies, colitis, cystitis, nervous stomach, constipation, etc.

Most of these are considered psychosomatic problems, at least in their origin. The moment at which a psychosomatic problem becomes a physical problem is a bit of a mystery but is generally considered to be that moment when the inflammation assumes a life of its own. I believe it is the moment when we label the discomfort the problem. For example, if my sinuses are bothering me, they may be "asking" me to eliminate a long term gnawing tension and to grab a better hold on myself with a vacation and a more restful work schedule. If I respond and the sinus condition goes away, I tell my friends I had a sinus infection. If I disregard the demands of my sinuses and merely irritate them with superficial sprays and medicines, it will not be long before I have a "*sinus condition*." Our bodies are amazingly accommodating. I may actually *want* the sinus condition to camouflage my psychosomatic problem. It is easier to blame my sinuses than to face the actual situation. And our body cooperates fully. It and I join together in a full dramatization of my sinusitis. By focusing our full attention on the "stricken area," we are able to develop a wonderful, self-perpetuating irritation that fully consumes all our emotional energies.

In too many cases we are advised to *learn to live* with our affliction. Drugs and a variety of nostrums are prescribed to merely make the problem bearable. This is not the case with those responsible doctors and psychiatrists who force us to seek out the underlying problem. For our purpose, for the self treatment of these ailments, we must ask ourselves, "what is the sinusitus *asking of me?*" We must probe the discomfort to receive its message.

The message of a constantly stuffed nose and aches behind the eyes may hardly seem that enlightening. Not so. If we concentrate on our whole feeling tone, we *do* find that the sinusitus is associated with an obsession, or a disappointment, or an unwillingness to fully involve our life force, or simple apathy. And deeper still, that the entire malaise is actually a plea from our wounded psyche, asking us to expend ourselves more fully, to fulfill ourselves as we were mysteriously meant to. If we do this, a genuine cure will be at hand. Otherwise our nature accommodates us in a perverse-positive way. We are given the opportunity to indulge the drama of destruction right to the hilt, even to a rapid annihilation of our life—self destruction without the overt act of suicide. This is a vital function of our nature. It is not a facetious act. It is the process of regeneration, nature devouring itself to recreate itself. The snake eating its tail. Our nature accommodates itself in all of its function.

High Blood Pressure

Some twenty-five million people suffer from high blood pressure in the United States alone. Of these, more than two thirds are referred to as cases of "essential hypertension," meaning that there is no organic cause for their problem—such as kidney infection or tumor. A battle is being waged between those who believe that this form of hypertension is due to stress—that it is a psychosomatic problem, and those who insist that it is a physiological problem that can be controlled chemically, but never cured. After years of intense study, the cause and certainly the cure of high blood pressure remains a mystery despite the fact that many regard it our number one killer.

It is generally agreed that the effect, not the cause, which creates the problem is constriction in the arteries which results from the contraction of the muscles in the arterial wall. It is also agreed that this occurs automatically when we are emotionally charged, due first to the nervous energy which the diencephalon exerts on the arterial muscles, and secondly to the release of adrenalin into the blood stream. The cause of this excitation can be modern life, family relationships, a psychological problem, fear, anxiety, diet, inherited characteristics.

The media keep warning us that we must regularly take our blood pressure. Their "not for profit" ads are terribly concerned about our health. But they let us know in the same breath that high blood pressure can be "controlled." What they mean is drug controlled and they seem to be more the agents of the drug companies (who can prove it?) than our guardian angels. They scare us half to death as they speak of the "silent killer" that causes heart seizure and stroke.

The notion that high blood pressure steals on us silently is sheer nonsense. The advent of high blood pressure is *anything but silent*. It rings a thousand bells loud and clear. The strain of overwork, the contraction of our bodies from lack of sleep, frustrated libido, a deep seated emotional problem, hyperactivity among children, the strain of excessive weight—all these and many more warning signs are letting us know that we are courting high blood pressure. We must ask ourselves if essential hypertension is a *condition* rather than a disease.

When the doctor finally observes the elevation of the needle that proclaims our high blood pressure, he is announcing a *cumulative* response to self-abuse. He is revealing a refusal to acknowledge our pain warnings. The slightest tension is made known to us immediately. That gnawing "hypertension" that we internalize as mild depression is as "vocal" as any other signal. If we do not respond, we are courting our own death. Our bodies are entirely accommodating. The contraction compounds until our blood flow, the feeding of each and every one of our trillions of cells and the will to live annihilate themselves in a cardio-vascular seizure. And the army of brilliant statisticians record such a death as a "coronary attack," as if it is a tragic accident, as if nature goofed, not the deceased.

How do we reverse this process? What can we do when it is far advanced? Doctors who utilize drugs to reduce the secretion of adrenalin, or block the brain action that excites the arterial rigidity, are dealing with the symptom, not the cause. The cause is revealed in anxiety pain, fear pain, depression pain, unhappiness pain. The cure is a complete reversal of our response patterns to pain. We must recognize that it is the healer, not the enemy.

Bio-feedback studies indicate that alpha waves tend to disappear as hypertension increases. This means that we are becoming mind responsive rather than *feeling responsive*, ultimately we go from one fearsome thought to another. I must act this or that way. I must be more spiritual, more aggressive, earn more money, improve my appearance, improve the appearance of my house, become an achiever, find an answer to every problem that besets me, exert absolute control over my circumstances, and so on ad infinitum without any trust in our innate wisdom or the function of our nature. This *must* lead to either physical or mental breakdown. High blood pressure may be the most common form of this breakdown.

It is very difficult to become calm, intuitive beings when we have fallen into this mind-centered cul-de-sac. We suffer tension that is unbearable. It is our inner self demanding a return to *trust in our inner self*, not to clutch at any single thing; to allow ourselves the luxury of total vulnerability, open heartedness, absence of constraint; an existence that is unqualified; a vascular system that is *self-disciplined* not mind distorted.

Most high blood pressure sufferers do not know where to start. Their minds are confused and tortured by outside advice and self doubt. They try to reduce their tensions but they are more tense than ever. It all suggests the fable of the ten blind men who touch an elephant and insist, by the experience of their touch, that an elephant is a tail, a trunk, a leg, a tusk and so forth. They cannot visualize the whole animal. Now imagine an elephant with a thousand different parts and we see the blind hypertension sufferer asking which foods to eat, which exercise to take, which attitudes to assume, which drugs to trust, which religion to observe. We have thousands of experts and thousands of options but how do we make the *correct choice*? What do we do from moment to moment?

Perhaps hypertension, as much as any other problem, illustrates the futility of trusting the *rational mind*. I am saying that correct choice must include instinct along with judgment. Our minds cannot sort out our needs from moment to moment, but our feelings *can*. Feelings can range through thousands of options and make a correct choice. They tell us *perfectly*, after we have exhausted our rational sanity. Direct response to pain and non-pain, to positive-negative feeling is an enormous aid to overcoming the high blood pressure problem. To sleep whenever we are sleepy; to reject activities that are displeasing and engage in activity that is pleasing; to respond to the slightest tension in the hand or foot; to feel good in family situations rather than to maintain the upper hand; to be absolutely comfortable in love rather than to be a hero in love; to trust our health and our future to our instinctive selves—this is the magic that no medicine and no advice can replace.

Severe Physical Illness

If we have proven that heart trouble or cancer among smokers is higher than among non-smokers, then we have equal proof that our failure to respond to smoker's cough, smoker's mouth and other smoking discomforts brings on these dread conditions. When does a case of emphysema or lung cancer start? Is it not the moment we take our first cigarette puff and the lungs complain with violent coughing? Does a stomach ulcer start when the bleeding begins, or when a slight stomach cramp pleads with us to stop stuffing our nervous stomach? Is weariness from persistent lack of sleep the first rudiment of a stroke? Is pain in our legs from overweight and lack of exercise the first sign of hardening of the arteries?

A minor heart attack brings a radical change in our habit patterns. We rest several months, stop smoking, drastically change our diet, take sensible exercise and call a decisive halt to all job and family stress. Our system has finally extracted a multiple response to years of multiple self damage. But an entire series of symptoms, shortness of breath, heart pains, palpitation, extreme nervousness, may only succeed in scaring us into an hour's sleep on a Sunday afternoon. How we delude ourselves until we take that frantic ambulance ride to the hospital!

Our mental and spiritual health deeply affects our physical health. If we feel the uncontrollable pain of loneliness, our nature is asking us to open ourselves to people, not to sit before a TV set weeks on end. If we have an uncomfortable sense of futility because we are cynical and purposeless, our nature is asking us to open ourselves up to our inner mystery and the mystery of all existence. This vast unknown constitutes ninety percent of our reality. The Hebrew word is *dereheretz*, respect for the unknown. The answer to futility is not heavy drinking or gambling or finding some means by which we can inflict torture on ourselves or others. There *is* some religious inquiry that will meet our need. And if nothing else works, a course in atomic physics or biology will quite adequately do the job.

Our amazing intuitive energy is constantly there, vibrating every second, a perfect servant, urging us on, showing us the way to avoid serious illness—to be attuned. Ultimately it attunes us to age and to death because these, also, are our *essential being*. But severe premature disease, half lives, depressed lives, will be enormously reduced when awareness and intuition rule our lives.

The time is approaching when we may regularly spend two or three weeks at an Instinct Attunement Center. Here, under the watchful eye of an entirely new breed of doctor-psychiatrist-religionist, we will re-attune ourselves *before* we become ill. This will be a hospital for the *well*. Concentration on our feeling-demands will return us to our essence. The staff and the bio-feedback instruments will be there to help us, but the essential job will be done *by us*.

We have the beginnings of such an approach today among a small group of healers who advocate a holistic approach to illness. These men and women attempt to prevent and to cure heart attack, cancer and all other severe illness by utilizing a multi-faceted approach. They cleanse the lungs with breathing exercises, they cleanse the encrusted intestines with various forms of enemas and with oils taken orally, they cleanse the blood stream and the inner body with fasting and diets of fresh, organic foods, they cleanse the organs and muscles with massage and yoga exercise, they cleanse the mind with meditation and chanting, they demand some spiritual commitment to cleanse cynicism and a new look at family and job entanglements to cleanse the emotions. They seek a new awareness of self, all this before they prescribe *any corrective action whatsoever*.

These same healers refuse to injure the body at the very moment they are healing the body. They seek to avoid surgery or radiation therapy for this reason. Though they prescribe drugs to help us live with our disease temporarily, they claim that drugs do not cure anything. Insulin does not cure diabetes. Antibiotics cannot cure infection unless the patient has enough natural resistance to remove the infection. They maintain that the body can heal itself if it is given a chance. After cleansing they prescribe sunlight, raw foods rich in enzymes and minerals, exercise, open hearted relationships and radical awe for the universe in which we live.

One Hundred Thousand Cures

Let us say that you missed the boat. You didn't anticipate the illness well enough to head it off. Now you are stuck with it. You are desperate to find a quick cure.

Do you leave it entirely to your doctor? I wouldn't—*not on my life.* Why should you—*on your life*? See your family doctor, *certainly*! See every possible specialist by all means. Do everything you possibly can. Surely if it is my body, *I owe it to myself to find out* all there is to know about my problem. I also believe that I am sensible enough to read the available literature. *Why shouldn't I* own a medical manual and seven or eight books that cover general fields such as "Back to Eden" by Jethro Kloss which reviews the natural healing methods employed by people for many centuries before medicine became the craft it is? There is also the local library and if necessary, a medical library in a nearby university. All these books have handy indices which quickly lead to available data. Does this make me an expert? Not at all. But *I can, I owe it to myself* to experiment with this data, and there is no fear whatsoever that I will harm myself, if I trust my being, and if I stay in touch with my *understanding* family doctor.

Let us take an example. Millions of men suffer urinary tract and prostatic problems. The pain this causes, the embarrassment, the actual loss of sexuality and the threat to self-confidence cannot be measured. Most of these men end up in the hands of a urologist. In almost every case he will prescribe antibiotics or other pills; he may suggest prostate massage; he will recommend eight or ten glasses of liquids a day; and he will advise abstinence from sex, liquor, coffee and spicy foods. In all likelihood, he will express the pious hope that the patient will avoid surgery. At this point—even without surgery—many men feel a sense of debilitating hopelessness as they trudge to their monthly visits with their urologist and wrestle with a kind of penis hypochondria. They are suffering gnawing and debilitating pain. What is this pain saying?

I believe this pain is asking for a new outlook. I believe it is asking for some self experimentation. Instead of becoming withdrawn and restricted, there should be an attempt to relaxation and well being. And spiritual openness will be a positive help. Executives and taxi drivers suffer this problem. They sit too much. Regular exercise is helpful. The natural healing books recommend a variety of antidotes. Heavy doses of vitamin C to cleanse the body, the zinc in pumpkin seeds and the acid in cranberry juice are recommended. Then there is self performed massage of the prostate by finger or certain yoga exercise and irrigation of the urethra with a catheter device, also self performed. Enemas, even high colonics, are highly recommended by those who insist there is a vital connection between the intestines and the urethral system. A more wholesome diet, more fresh air, meditation to quiet the nerves, tranquilizers for a few days, and intensified sexual activity after the immediate symptoms are removed may also help.

Do any of these suggestions interfere with the recommendations of your doctor? Can they do anything but help? Are you betraying or helping yourself? Will your signals—pain or relief from pain—misdirect you if you are careful to check with your doctor about the presence of infection in your urine? Or if you have any doubts, do you have the *right to ask* your doctor about combining these self assisting remedies with your doctor's recommendations? *Of course you do*!

Fifteen years ago the medical profession disdained psychosomatic factors, nutrition and viruses as possible causes of cancer. Today the medical establishment is spending millions researching these areas. The "quacks," the "charlatans" of those days who concerned themselves with these matters are no longer disparaged. To trust ourselves without mistrusting the experts is no sin. It may save our lives. It is our joyous privilege and our duty.

If there is no crime in allowing our feelings and our impulses to aid in the choice of doctors and techniques, there is also no crime in the use of more esoteric forms of healing such as psychic, faith and naturopathic healing. Who can deny that there is an extraordinary intelligence in nature? Who has the right to deny us the more adventuresome, more optimistic frame of mind which comes from feeling that no problem is an insurmountable problem? It is the hard-nosed scientist who may be *most* inaccurate because he restricts treatment to proven fact which totals no more than five percent of ultimate scientific truth.

There are natural healers and psychic healers today who combine the latest scientific instruments and their own perceptive capacities with amazing accuracy. To seek them out, to exploit this merger of the psychological, the physical, and the metaphysical, is both a legitimate and an inspiring experience.

Chapter Seven

EMOTIONAL IMBALANCE

All of us are besieged by some degree of emotional pain. A lingering sense of malaise, mild depression, feeling bound by a situation, a masochistic attachment, anxiety, unnecessary hostility, nervousness, fear.

More often than not, we are aware that the emotional pain has no rational basis. But we can't throw it off, no matter how unfounded or ridiculous it is. At times, the more we try, the more it persists.

Our normal procedure is to try to *reason* the difficulty away. Our minds are hard at work on a number of theories. We try this or that approach. We reach into our childhood for a psychological explanation. We try a spiritual solution. A friend or a book sparks an entirely new idea. We fight our malaise. It remains the "enemy." If we fail to overcome the "enemy" over any length of time, we label ourselves *neurotic*.

At no time do we *accept* the malaise. At no time do we consider the possibility that this "enemy" may actually be a friend. Most of us never dream that every pang of emotional pain has a positive purpose. We spend months theorizing over the problem, without ever taking a moment to look to the *pain itself* for guidance.

Let us say that two people are suffering from long-term anger. It may be directed at a husband, wife, lover, child, parent, fellow worker. They have tried every possible solution: discussion, argument, compromise, psychological help, prayer, temporary separation, and fury.

Nothing has solved the problem. The anger continues unabated. Both antagonists are convinced they are absolutely right, logically, philosophically, lawfully, and in the eyes of whatever god they worship. We have all seen people methodically destroy each other in the name of *reason*. Reason will never solve the issue. In the name of reason, we can take one hundred different "iron clad" stands on any issue.

Suppose we take time to meditate on the *anger pain itself*. Suppose we completely forget every single technicality, every fine point. Perhaps you want to try it. Take a few minutes to think of a personal situation. Think of that individual who makes your hackles rise in anger. Perhaps it is a person from whom you separated some time ago. Try to completely forget who was right and who was wrong, who *did* this and who *did* that. Instead, examine or reconstruct your feelings, the ache in your heart. Do it now.

Did the feeling you experienced deep in the pain shed any light on the argument? Do you have a broader acceptance of the argument now? Do you wonder why the situation affected you so severely?

If we review *our feelings* about the anger rather than its fine technicalities, we find we don't take it too seriously. We are left with an impression that can hardly be put into words. We somehow *know* that the situation is a game that has been carried to ridiculous extremes. We *know* that we *must allow* the situation to take care of itself, that we can trust—and ultimately *will trust* ourself to our future self. Perhaps this core feeling will tell us to take a forthright action, to take extreme action—perhaps to cease the relationship. But the decision is now absolutely correct. It did not come from inferior *mind logic*. It came from *feeling logic*. This decision may force a laugh out of us, or draw a tear. It will be beyond further questioning.

All of us confuse emotion with feeling. Emotion is intuitive feeling mixed with thought. It is an attempt to *hold on* to intuitive feeling, to bottle it, whereas intuitive feeling rises out of each and every moment. (In Hindu thought, it *is* the moment.) It takes no great effort to exaggerate any emotion to the point of paranoia or hysteria with the "help" of thought. And yet, if we *stay with* the feeling, *stay with* the pain, all our emotional pain will *dissolve itself*. The one is emotional imbalance, the other is the magnificent function of this collective nature. Too many psychologists will claim that this is gross *oversimplification*. I am afraid that they are addicted to *over complication*.

Pain blindness and feeling blindness is the cause of most of the emotional illness and mass hysteria of our age. It is not the atom bomb that will destroy our civilization—our over indulged thought minds are already doing the job too efficiently. Our presumptuous cortex minds are eroding our entire diencephalic-autonomic systems by keeping us in a perpetual state of anxiety. This physical damage plus the hatred, the rage with which we react to our seeming disorder, is making us all enemies to ourselves and to each other.

We all have sudden moments when our emotional being appears to cure itself spontaneously. An amazing clarity unites body, mind, feeling. Conjecture is replaced by an instinctual absolute. At this point we *know* and we know that we know. There is no longer a single false move. We feel no emotional imbalance.

Sleeplessness

Sleeplessness is a curse. There are few irritations as frustrating as desperate search for sleep. The antidotes to sleeplessness run into the thousands. Herbs, warm milk, exercise, pleasant thoughts, body relaxation, drugs, counting sheep, a vacation and so on. These may help to a greater or lesser degree. Certainly a happy, normal life, a decent job, rest, exercise, help enormously. But what can we do when some physical or mental perversity keeps us awake? What do we do when the more we strive for sleep, the more it eludes us?

Sleep must will *itself*. We cannot command sleep. We cannot impose our voluntary self on the involuntary process of falling asleep. We are better off *forgetting* about our sleeplessness.

But by now we are irritated by our irritation. This causes a chain reaction. Sleeplessness aggravates sleeplessness. By now we tell ourselves that for tonight, at least, we have a case of insomnia. This *intensifies* our irritation and we are off to the races: self-castigation, anger, crazy attempts to impose sleep, a panorama of torture.

There is an alternative. First, we must determine that we will impose *nothing* on ourselves. *Not one antidote*. To execute one single remedy is to cling to a voluntary act *which is opposite to the involuntary state of sleep*. Instead of trying to fight off each irritation, we must let them come as they will; we must allow them to *tell us*. Whatever irritation presents itself of its own accord *is involuntary. We are far closer to the involuntary state of sleep*.

If we do not try to fight off the tension in the hand or back or shoulder region, we will respond to these precise requests for changes in our body position. If we do not mask the hostility we feel over a business conflict, the pain in the hostility will present the situation in a sensible perspective. If we do not try to disregard the emotional anxiety that causes pain in our heart region, we will find that this same pain is pushing us to relieve this anxiety and to react to the tension that causes it. If my mind is tortured with thought, this same pain is showing the way to release from this torture. If we are assaulted by abject thoughts, it is better to go right down to the core of our miserable feeling—not to deny that there are many aspects of our life experience that are totally bleak—better to *feel* this bleakness without any sugar coating or rationalization. Somehow it becomes a cleansing process. The inner being, the inner brain takes over and we fall asleep.

If the mind still remains perverse, examine the *pain of the perversity*. No antidotes, no remedies, as stated before, except to follow the dictates of the pain. Our instinctive being does not resist sleep, it irrevocably pursues sleep. If we quit trying to help it—allow it to call the signals—we will be amazed at the speed with which *it* puts us to sleep. These pain states derive from our instinctive being. They bring on sleep automatically.

In Oriental philosophy, the state of dreamless sleep is considered the *actual state* of our being. The cortex stops functioning. We are in the hands of our absolute being, undisturbed by the meddling mind. With amazing proficiency, the brain stem, the autonomous nervous system, each organ, each and every cell, join to restore our physical, mental and emotional being.

Public and Social Nervousness

Nervousness wrecks the careers of many performers. Almost all of us, including seasoned performers, are clutched by intense fears that sometimes border on insanity. Walk into any theatre, concert hall, sports locker room, lecture hall, before a performance and you will find sweating, jumpy, cursing, miserable performers. The adrenalin is pouring. A perverse internal ogre is insisting they are about to face indecent exposure—or total paralysis.

Successful performers do a great job despite the nervousness. Others fall apart. These label themselves permanent victims of stage fright. Ultimately many give up promising careers.

Many performers tell us that nervousness is helpful. The adrenalin sharpens their reflexes. And the fear—the pain of the fear is a *rapid fire warning system* that sharpens the performance. If it is examined carefully, the nervousness is actually opposite to compulsive fear.

Perhaps the best speaker I have ever known amazed an audience when he announced the secret of his enormous ability. "I make it a point," he declared, "never to think about the subject of a pending lecture for as much as a week or two in advance. I refuse to be burdened with a single phrase or idea that inhibits my thinking process *during* the lecture. It doesn't allow me to be spontaneous, to sense the thinking of the audience, to allow the vast capacities of my intuitive nature to reach into wonderful new areas. It deprives me of a rhythm and cadence which is as vital to the presentation as the subject material."

Such speakers *share* any difficulty they have with the audience. The very fact that they express their doubts to the audience, fits right into the subject matter. It brings the audience into the speaker's confidence. Everything is right if it is freely expressed—within the relative moment. This is the majesty of our existence.

The identical factors enter into our social performance. We have thousands of books that advise us how to improve our social behavior. Most of these systems provide "how to" instructions that *stand between* us and our instinct by becoming a false crutch. Even one such crutch destroys our spontaneity. Nowhere do we find the suggestion that direct discomfort reaction is the surest guide to an outgoing personality. If you observe yourself for any length of time, you discover that your "nature" wants you to be at ease, blissfully happy at all times. This may sound corny and false. Read the message of your social discomforts and be amazed.

So many of us hide our self-consciousness under some camouflage. We become jokesters, compulsive careerists, or world saviors. We present an *assumed image* of ourselves to the world. Ultimately our ambivalence makes us tongue-tied or forces us to say things we do not wish to say. Is this inadequacy or is it fury at ourselves for *not being ourselves*? An inner voice is screaming at us. "Stop being diffident! Stop running off at the mouth. Stop being such a hero! Trust the moment. Trust yourself! *Be* yourself! Why should you fear anyone?"

"Very well," we may say. "I *want* to be myself, but I want to be interesting and casual and lively and comfortable. Do I have everything I need, the background, the training, the ability?" Yes you have EVERYTHING! *Everything you require*! The precise moment that you are being yourself, your intuition tells you that you are being yourself. The moment that you are standing on your own two feet, born of our common nature and an equal to anyone in the world, there are no pain messages. When you are not demeaning yourself, (creating your own *karma*) you are floating on an effortless, intuitive vibration that is doing it all for you. Any difficulty you feel becomes a topic of discussion. You are open, free to express whatever comes to mind. Not canned material that you have delivered a thousand times; this freezes conversation. Just whatever comes out of the wavelength. And it is all there, even if it is nothing more than a nod or a giggle.

Anxiety, Excitability, Depression

There is a type of emotional difficulty that feeds on itself. The problem intensifies the problem. Anxiety creates its own anxiety. Excitability creates its own excitability. Ultimately these lead to depression which then creates its own depression. These self-generating, repeater neuroses create a separate person within our person, what psychiatry calls a split personality. Let us take depression as our example.

To a greater or lesser degree, depression has become a universal malaise. We take it to be normal and inevitable. We consider it perfectly acceptable for a person to be entirely dependent on liquor or pot or six hours a day of TV, or an entirely cynical attitude to get through the day. There are many circles in which a smiling face or a happy voice is a threat—actually held in contempt. The "correct" presence is a clouded face, an irascible and molested nature. Unhappy is *in*. Happy is out. Pleasure is restricted to the sharing of mutual displeasure with other depressives. It is "okay" to enjoy relationships with children up to two years of age and dogs. Even love and sex are passé. The general atmosphere is becoming so bad that anyone not already depressed is rapidly becoming a depressive.

But depression is no superficial matter. Depression is

wasting millions of lives. It is driving other millions to a perverse, hateful, bizarre existence. Fashionable or not, it is a devastating experience. An unexplained uneasiness hangs over our head. Much of the time we are depressed without any notion as to why we are depressed.

If we attempt to overcome the depression with thought—with our minds—we are beset with unbearable confusions. Which of several psychiatric theories should we apply to the depression? Is the depression caused by guilt, by a prideful need for self-image, by a family condition, by spiritual emptiness, by sexual repression, by job or money frustration, by some accidental misunderstanding? "Why do I *suffer* this depression, am I a depressive?"

Depression will persist indefinitely—it will feed voraciously on its own cursed self until we discover that the *pain* of depression has a vital purpose, *to rid us of the depression.* Our endless theorizing about what originates the depression causes us to misinterpret this pain. We think the pain is the culprit when actually its purpose is to *oppose* the depression, to *rid us* of it, to recognize its *absurdity*.

If we stop theorizing and mulling and ask ourselves, "What is this *depression pain* asking of me?" we obtain an automatic result. The pain is insistently demanding that we give up this absurdity. If we *feel* the pain to our core, it immediately tunes us into our life force. A wonderful feeling of contentment envelops us. When this life force is flowing, our contentment is absolute, unquestioned and unending. It is not a thought contentment, "I am content because I just bought my family an automatic pop corn dispenser and *I should be* content." (Deep down we know the dispenser will some day break, it will cause fights, it will gather dust.) I am merely content in my *aliveness.* I am content because my pain message restored my sanity, because it *is* my sanity.

How, you may ask, does this work? If we examine feelings closely—if we examine our pains closely—we discover that they are far more astute than thought. A feeling can hardly be put into words. It contains so much more than words can describe. Words and thought simply cannot manage the infinite complexity of our situations. Feelings encompass these intricacies and their solutions.

The pain of shame is designed to rid us of shame. The pain of guilt is designed to rid us of guilt. The pain of frustration is designed to help us to see beyond our frustration. The pain of being bullheaded is designed to help us see things in their longer term. If we suffer from the pain of excitability or panic or sadness or misery, we find that this pain is not meant to exaggerate these states. Just the opposite! The purpose of the pain is to mollify these states, to return us to our aliveness. The pain itself *is* our aliveness! It is our nature and the collective eternal nature —perfect despite its seeming imperfection.

This process requires experimentation. Instead of searching for a thousand solutions and finding no solutions, we must gradually induce the wisdom of the pain to automatically handle itself. It will not fail us. It will tell us what wants doing—where to defer to a situation and where to assert ourselves.

Most of our neuroses are saying, "Hey, you are missing the point! You are missing the point of your existence. Your neurosis *is not* plaguing you, it is your inner self *crying out that it does not want to be plagued*. Every discomfort suggests a pre-condition; it points to a pre-existent state of absolute *comfort*. This essential design, or life field, or Atman as the yogis call it, is our actual being. It is constantly readjusting and returning our being to the electromagnetic concept that was expressed in our first ovum-sperm. It is a biologic as well as an etheric reality. This perfect, unlimited, unqualified Atman self is filled with pleasure, joy, humor as well as a good bit of mad absurdity. Does this sound inconceivable, corny? Respond to your emotional imbalance, do not mask it, before you make your judgment.

CHAPTER EIGHT

MENTAL DIFFICULTY

Mental difficulty abounds. I am referring to difficulty in decision making; should I take a job, should I enter a business, what career will give me satisfaction, how should I deal with my spouse, with my child, which of several plans should be utilized for a project?

On the face of it, it would seem absurd that spontaneous instinct can somehow invade the area of simple reason. We tend to think that any practical problem must be confronted with facts and figures. Certainly the totals that show on an IBM sales print-out should tell us more about a marketing problem than sheer intuition. It would seem so. Yet our world has never had more facts and figures at its disposal and has never seemed more at sea politically, economically, healthwise, emotionally. In recent years, our machines and our computers have been racing ahead of us. They have a life of their own and our most essential needs are being disregarded.

Let us take an everyday example. A man contemplates a change of job. He must measure about a hundred separate factors: salary, relocation, friends, schools, associates, advancement, cultural facility, recreational facility, religious facility, cost of a new house, price for the old house, a large number of similar questions relative to his wife and children, etc. Can he arrive at a true answer?

Unless there is some overriding factor—a fifty percent rise in salary—his decision will be an agonizing hassle. His mind will be in a state of juggling turmoil for months. It may seem that no objective choice is possible. Yet if he stops figuring and deeply examines his feelings, he may discover that he simply must remain because he and one associate are attuned to each other, or he must leave because he and one associate have a subtle mistrust of each other. The state of his prevailing mental health must be the decisive factor. All other factors will fade out of contention. So that the intuitive logic of the pain feeling has sorted out this "impossible problem" with infinitely more capacity than his adding machine mind.

Another example. Let us say that I am a housewife who has been holding a job for a number of years. A younger woman in the firm is telling management that she wants my job. I could cry out in horror that I need the job to help sustain my family and to keep occupied. Or I could tell myself that I *have been* contemplating giving my full time to my family. My husband and my children try to help me reconcile myself to losing the job, and several friends give me a hundred reasons which absolutely prove that giving up the job would be a surrender to weakness.

Again I can agonize to a point bordering on madness. But if I examine my feelings, I may find that all the issues—justice, seniority, friends in management, money, health—do not add up to a fig. My feeling intuition is telling me that my deepest ache is concern for my husband. He has worked on one job for thirty years and it has become a threat to his mental and physical health. It is time for me and my husband to prepare for a creative change, to settle on a farm in a rural atmosphere.

The entire world is being strangled by so called "*reason*." National reason, military reason, political reason, economic reason, advertising reason, and religious reason. But reason and expediency have become interchangeable words. There was a time when reason was equated with higher instinct, with conscience—words that are in general disrepute today. Insatiable desire for a pizza pie is considered the ultimate experience of instinct. Conscience is confused with false guilt. The net result is loss of an entire spectrum of cognitive awareness, to say nothing of the loss of affection and civility. Bottom line reason is literally depriving us of our souls.

We *must* believe that mental agonizing comes from decisions that are being attempted on a strict *quid pro quo* basis—that the pain is "demanding" consideration for our *collective being*, our *collective society*. Not as a duty to this or that religious or ethical code, but as a duty to *our own and our collective instinct*.

Decision making can be agonizing even in the most mundane matters. A young man may be bordering on compulsive insanity because he can't choose one of a dozen different makes of compact cars. He insists that his agony lies in the complicated relative merits of the various cars. But does it? His pain is actually telling him to make a choice; to enjoy this fantastic vehicle that will allow him to range the world, whichever car he chooses. His pain is telling him he is demeaning this miracle by debating rear window wipers versus twenty square feet of trunk space.

If we meditate briefly on the pain we suffer, rather than the problem, we find that even decision making is an intuitive process. Our inner computer is unbelievably accurate if we don't gum up the works with memory references. If you have doubts, try this process with any business or practical problem. You will be amazed.

Chapter Nine

SPIRITUAL ANGUISH

Mankind's greatest frustration may be the notion that we must go through endless ritual and dogma before we can feel order in our universe. All of us search for some sign which will confirm purpose and sanity in our existence, which will reveal the secret of all secrets. We place our heads and hearts in the hands of any person or belief that promises *the answer*. We are prepared to make any vow, any resolution, any sacrifice to explain this mad world. But time and again we feel cheated by religious blandness, by hocus pocus, by spiritual materialism. Still we do not stop. The search haunts us for a lifetime. Again and again we find an ineffable beauty in this universe. Our hopes are raised. But then we see the suffering on one city street, or read of a mass catastrophe, or lower our eyes at the signs of encroaching age on the face of a friend, and we are thrust into a trough of despair.

All religions do not hesitate to proclaim that God or Godhood is *within us*. If this is so, how can we explain our massive spiritual anguish? Why does nature withhold its secret so jealously? Does this universe really *have* an ultimate secret?

The "still, small voice" within us is not a mystery in Eastern philosophy. It *is there* each and every second. It is our instinctive being, this intimate *I*—this awareness of self—this often dissolute, puzzled *I* that we are so quick to put down. It is this very I-ness that feels and thinks and hurts and sees and hears and questions and laughs and cries. These Eastern saints, or are they madmen, insist that this *collective I-ness creates our natural law, creates the world and creates the universe*! Is this possible—remotely conceivable? Are all the natural laws of the universe *our doing*? Is the vast scientific absolute—every atom, every neutron—something that *we devised*?! Is it beyond sanity to believe that life rises from life, that the collective existence rises from the collective existence? Where do we find even the *vaguest* intimation that this is true? By what smidgen of evidence can we believe this? By trusting existence, say the mystics. By permitting our own spiritual discomfort to guide us to spiritual comfort, just as we trust all the vast physical forces in nature to ultimately exist in absolute equilibrium. By perceiving that our life experience is a universally derived experience in addition to being a personal experience. By observing that we comprise one omni-psychology; that cognition, mentation, instinct, love, hate, sexuality, pleasure, pain are an encompassing reality—a vast world beyond the limited perception of our minds—but *our world*!

We speak of achieving God's *grace*. In the East they speak of the *Supreme Guru within*. In both cases religionists tell us that this involuntary process is required if we are to find a higher reality. If they are correct, how do we become spiritually involuntary? How do we pierce through vanity, ego, intellectuality, mind, instinct—to REALITY? And what will happen if we do?

I cannot tell you. It must be a matter of experience between you and your inner self, between you and your instinctive process. There is nothing mystical about this. When we wake in the morning from deep, dreamless sleep, we are remarkably attuned. We feel cleansed, restored, blissful, transported by an array of exquisite feelings and day dreams. We have somehow solved our most difficult problems—for a few minutes we are at peace with the world. This state came to us *involuntarily*—through the most inactive capacity that had nothing to do with our conscious intent—through sleep.

But then our eyes move to the clock which announces our rise and shine time and a stentorian voice proclaims, "All further sweet feelings must *cease*! You must rise and assume your inner and outer mask. Any such happiness throughout the day is forbidden with the following exceptions:

1. You can be high on alcohol or drugs.

2. Celebration of an occasion such as a birthday or anniversary may rouse limited feeling.

3. The sweet smell of success fantasy is fully authorized.

4. Sexual fantasy is fine, but excessive sexual pleasure is a no-no.

5. You may briefly adore a flower, a dog, a child, a loved one, or God provided that you are intensely aware of the privilege which is being accorded to you."

The mysterious vibration that we feel as we rise, sustains every blade of grass, every tree, every bird, every living thing. If we deny ourselves this Alpha wave, or ultimate contentment wave, or life force wave, we are miserable. We become blamers. We blame ourselves and each other and we hate ourselves and each other for this misery.

Is it possible to augment such morning contentment for an hour, for a full day, for a month—in all our activities —in work, in love, in the tiring chores of the day? Is it possible to be in an almost permanent state of grace? Is this our *actual* state, and is all spiritual anguish, spiritual pain demanding a return to that spiritual center in which we find absolute reason in all things? Is pain the means by which our pure being returns itself to pure being? Finally, is this pure being—this constant emanation—an endless beginning in which we have played and will play an eternal role?

The Yogic and Buddhist literature repeat a hellishly perplexing phrase which reads, "There is no suffering, no sickness, no death." Can you imagine a more irritating, presumptuous assertion? What they mean is that suffering is a process. That it is *ridding* us of attachment to our unilateral self and is therefore non-existent. Even if this is so, how can they go on to assert that sickness and death are likewise non-existent? They insist that these too are a life process—an evolutionary process—a process not a state. They assert that meditative examination of the feelings that support this process will reveal that our legitimate state is nothingness—Godhood—Consciousness—design—omnipresence—omnipotence—omniscience. But once again I am exceeding the limits of this volume. Only intuitive grasp of our reality can confirm or deny this.

Meditation and Prayer

There are any number of meditative and prayer techniques. Many seekers stand in absolute adoration before the indescribable life force, or before a divine figure such as Christ, Buddha or Mohammed. Others seek only to perform "God's will" in absolute humility, by serving mankind. Occultists search for powers. Mystics dive for pearls of truth. But at heart, all these techniques are designed to bring us to a state of grace, to an involuntary state of pure being, to a reality that transcends our games.

The scriptures insist that such a reality exists *within us*. It is our prior condition. If this is so, isn't there some way by which we can respond to this prior condition without getting wound up in dogmas, words, ideas, theories, confusions? Isn't every feeling *somehow related* to this prior condition? Let us see if it is. Let us discharge words and theories from our minds. Let us allow our spiritual discomforts to state their own case. Are they *bringing* us to our absolute spiritual self, or are they declaring our spiritual inadequacy? Those who pray or meditate receive moments of extraordinary insight or grace. Do these moments come because of some special effort or technique, or do they rise *automatically* when we allow our spiritual despairs to help rather than hinder us?

Answer this question yourself. Is it possible that the feeling that is at the core of each spiritual difficulty is actually showing you the way to solve the difficulty? If you allow your involuntary self to function, if you respond to the pain feeling, are these discomforts raising you to a higher and higher state of spiritual equilibrium and perception? You may wish to experiment with this a moment, to allow your inner heart, your inner voice, your inner mind go to wherever it is they wish to go.

Did you find that your rational mind tends to block your release to spiritual surrender? This is to be expected. The ego mind is loath to give up its precious rights and privileges. But did you also find that your feelings are stronger than your rational mind? Let us meditate again. This time *allow* the blocks and conundrums which your rational mind poses to come forward. Go deep into the pain that is incited by these blocks. You may discover that each block somehow catapults you to a state of greater clarity. The pain caused by the block wants to eliminate that very block. Ultimately the instinctive state is discovered to be *our absolute state, our prior condition*.

Many, for whom this is a radical experience, will say that prayer is a dialogue with God, that God is an external being whose effulgent light we only faintly reflect. They will insist that there is no relationship with God except in an atmosphere of humble worship. This is a false boundary according to Eastern philosophy and to our own Judeo-Christian mystic tradition which holds that it is possible to *worship* and at the same time to *be* the incredible Life Force.

The more we are beleaguered by spiritual anguish, the more this pain *demands* response. But we are being asked to respond to spiritual pain intuitively, *not* to canned theories that we have been regurgitating for years and years. If prayer and meditation only seek a higher, more elite, holier than thou state, the result is synthetic. We are inevitably slapped down by this form of patronizing worship. Our own consciousness rejects it.

But our God-Godhood nature will bring us to the highest state imaginable if our prayer and meditation is rooted in the joys and sorrows of our real-life. Suddenly it all makes sense as things are—*as it is*—not on some idealistic, surrealistic plane. This explains the often higher wisdom and perception of so-called plain people. Ultimately, the most devastating life experiences, the most abject despair, the most impossible conundrum bottoms out and all people gain a glimpse of the "truth that surpasseth human understanding."

What a wonderful paradox! Our spiritual ascetics place themselves above the pain of reality and lose the very truth to which they devote their entire lives. And the plain people—street people, jokers, unsophisticates—who aspire to nothing but the drama and tumble of life, touch truth without any effort. And between these "highest" and "lowest" states, everybody is equally close to truth. Pain balances the spiritual scale perfectly no matter where we find our heads and hearts.

Terminal Illness, Death and Bereavement

Ultimately we all die. Ultimately old age or terminal illness undermines our health. Ultimately we lose those we love and suffer the unbearable pain of bereavement. Does this most excruciating of all pain have anything to offer us? What answer is there—what surcease is there for incurable illness, for the oblivion of death?

The sages speak of an afterlife, or of reincarnation. They offer quotes from the scriptures. They make complex deductions. Most of these statements are too subtle for general understanding.

Those who face a terminal disease or have survived an extreme emergency tell us that extreme pain, the experience of absolute hopelessness leaves them with a very special wisdom. A new truth stands fully revealed to them. Is this rationalization? Is this the simple fact of surrender? Or does the pain itself, unadorned by speculation, transmit its unmistakable perception?

What is this wisdom? In Vedantic philosophy and in Judeo-Christian mysticism, aging exists but not age, dis-ease exists but not disease, dying exists but not death. The first are all processes, the second are static states. Perhaps this is best illustrated if we meditate on our self ravaging process. We and all creatures decay and die. Is this the inevitable wear and tear of existence? Or is this our own essential process—*our nature* devouring itself to regenerate itself? Those who revolt with anger and disgust, only succeed in accelerating the process. Those who watch the irrevocable toll of our days and years, who "join in" with the inevitability of it, whose feeling sensors remain open, perceive that *they* are death itself (the process) in addition to being that which is dying. They are sickness itself (the process) as well as that which is sick. The message of their pain (do not take my word for it—experience this yourself) is that dying is not death and aging is not age, and even living is not life. The message is that our true nature is process—we are *both* creator and created. We are unending *creation*, rising constantly out of each and every moment, out of *ourselves*.

If we meditate further on this pain-process we may sense that no outside force *condemns* us to terminate our existence; that it is actually *our* conscious or superconscious choice. Our equilibrium requires death for its perfect function.

If we intensify this awareness even further, we find there is another, more frightening intimation. Our gaze falls directly on the fact that we have undeniable inclinations to destroy other people and to destroy ourselves. There is a piranha streak in our nature that is evidenced in envy, heartlessness, disdain, preoccupation with our self-image, a fascination with violence. We have been told that this is an evolutionary characteristic that derives from our fight for survival. But Vedic thinking carries this a step further.

The Orientals call this vicious streak our Kali nature, named after the killer goddess Kali who represents that aspect of our existence that dances with joy in burial grounds, at the burning ghat, wherever there is catastrophe. Our piranha-like aspect *wants* our death and *wants* the death of others. It is *we*, the Vedics insist, who are destroying our life to create our life. It is our higher consciousness shedding its collective skin—a daily process of dying and birthing. It is the fashion in our society to recoil from this reality, to deny its very existence. Kali worshippers in India say, "If you wish to see the *power* of our God or Godhood—see how inexorably our nature devours itself." They urge us to face and examine this pain and misery. It is the expenditure of our collective being, of our being's being. As the Easterners put it, without this expenditure, all of nature (Godhood itself) would atrophy and wither away from lack of use. Our collective being requires this activity, this jazz of life, this vast phantasmagoria to energize itself. It is our game, our joy, our pathos, our playground, our love, and our collective absurdity.

It would seem that nothing is as overwhelming as the loss of a loved person. How inconceivable that a precious body is forever locked away in the earth to decay and become nothing. At our funeral rites we shed inconsolable tears and feel that nothing remains for us in this insensitive cosmos.

But then, every bereavement is also a catharsis. The pain is also a cleansing. Wakes, and family togetherness following a funeral are accompanied by a certain inexplicable renewal. We somehow sense, or even enjoy the reality of that inner being that destroys itself to recreate itself. We *do* intimate a higher reason. Something soothes us. Time and again people say it is the soul of the departed that is comforting us. What they are saying, is that *there is some baffling mystery in the pain, that balances the terror.*

Severe and terminal sickness also has a liberating function. Deep down, something within us does not mind at all, in fact enjoys the prospect of *packing it in, the whole mess*! Our most impossible pain from injury or sickness carries the banner of *ultimate reality*. We are finally down to rock truth.

Our pain may also tell us that even our sense of futility and cynicism has its purpose. Hindus call this the whip of Shiva. Our nature whips us to make something of our days—to expend our lives for a burning political cause, or the search for some elusive invention, or an artistic will-o'-the-wisp. If we do not, Shiva's whip—our inevitable emptiness—will cause our self-destruction. Our nature is remorseless with itself. It allows us no quarter. If we limit the worth of the universe to the needs of our *personal* survival, we become irritable and fragile. If we refuse to couple the mundane with the supramundane, we feel automatic despair. And so it goes.

So each and every discomfort *does have* its message and its function. And it is this law, this omni-psychology which is the Consciousness or Godhead of which the Yogis speak. The whole of this law, the whole of nature exists in every living thing and in all of matter. The laws of its change are unchanging—despite the constant change. This is the perpetual reality. We each carry the total Godhood within ourselves, just as each of our trillions of cells carries our total body within it. So that all of being, the entire universe, rises from, is maintained by and returns to life, to us. We are simultaneously the part and the whole of the universe. We perceive and transcend our nature by *responding* to it, not by trying to transcend it. It is not our relationship with ourselves that matters nor our relationship with others, nor with nature, nor even with God or Godhood. It is the fact that all these relationships are absolute—beyond assessment or relationship. And pain, as we learn if we observe it, is the leveler that constantly returns us to our unwavering reality.

All this was once pronounced insane by scientists. Today the laws of relativity and quantum physics, the awesome power of the atom have drawn scientists to a new look at this godless Godhood theology. Just as we cannot perceive what it is to be a ray of light moving from the sun to the earth, or electricity travelling through miles of circuit instantly, or a TV signal that covers every speck of the earth, so our minds cannot perceive that very force *by which we are*. We do not *see* the electricity in a hot wire. We certainly *feel it*. Similarly, we do not see our reality, but we do feel it.

Spiritual realization is not limited to a private club. And we are not required to be absurd slaves to holy men or obscure scripture in order to obtain applications to this club. This is the most heartless conspiracy in all the history of mankind. Not only do we have the keys to the kingdom, but we live in the kingdom—and we *are* the kingdom!

Some will argue that this philosophy gives people the license to parade as God, to become bizarre, fanatical, destructive. The contrary is true. Those who perceive the self consuming role of nature are *not* aroused to the same destructive bitterness which is felt by many who despair over our seeming futility. *Apres moi le deluge*! If *I am* that magnificent open ended totality, it requires no outside force or fear to make me open, loving, peaceful. It is not a shaky obligation born out of *assumed* moral or religious principles. My love and consideration for my own life and the lives of others is automatic.

Chapter Ten

LOVE AND SEXUAL FRUSTRATION

How many people back away from a fulfilling love and sex life?

Why do so many love relationships turn to ashes and to hate?

Why is sexual failure the most prevalent cause of love failure at a time when sexual openness and honesty are supposed to be at an all time high?

Is it a fact that time *must diminish* love?

What prayer, what love potion, what remedy can rekindle love and desire when these appear to be dead?

Can love be endlessly renewed?

The desire for love and coitus is universal. Fulfilling relationships should be the privilege of every man and woman. Our instinctive self flowers in tumescence. Nobody should be deprived of enormously comfortable, long lasting, profoundly meaningful sex.

Our instinct pursues perfection in love and sexuality as relentlessly as it seeks physical and emotional equilibrium. There are a number of cultures in the East where sex is considered a sacrament, as sacred as prayer. We touch indescribable heights in fulfilled love. The experience carries us to states that far transcend our rational mind and for days afterward, all is somehow *right with the world.*

To be totally surrendered to the ultimate sexual experience is to touch the universal nature in which we all reside. A man and woman want desperately not so much to satisfy themselves or each other, as to achieve a third state which is beyond time, space, measurement or comprehension. Is it any wonder that we fantasize sex so continuously, that our drive for love refuses to be denied? Unfulfilled love causes extreme pain. Does this pain indicate an inferior person, sexual inadequacy, some mysterious psychological ailment? Should it be the signal for despair, self hate, sexual paralysis? Or should it be a tremendous catalyst, the motor power for greater maturity? Is fear of sexual inadequacy a *demand* from our psyche for a profound and fulfilling experience? Are sexual inhibitions actually a cry from our deepest heart for a new plateau of ecstatic experience? Is the anger and jaded sadism of contemporary sex, *rejection* of the short order love we serve up to ourselves today?

Love is not a unilateral experience. It requires the willing participation of two people. If either one is not fully responsive, the relationship will fail. Love and desire cannot depend on will. We cannot fake the giving or the receiving of love. Our minds may be temporarily deceived but our hearts and our genitals are *never* deceived. They reject the relationship.

What is the source of genuine desire? And how can it be maintained? The answer is less a mystery than we make it. To love, to open our heart and being to another person is not simply to find pleasure from the other person. It is a sharing of some mysterious universal vibration with that person. We love an entertainer, we love a child or parent, we love a sports hero, we love a religious or political leader when these individuals touch a chord in our deepest being. It is not simply an exchange for services rendered. It is the capacity to motivate that mysterious flow of being that inhabits all of us. It is the force that breaks through our self-conscious, constricting mind and reaches our instinctive, non-rational reality. We are always totally alive to that force. A child's innocence never fails to move us; a lover's tears, a friend's confusion, a tragi-comic situation crashes through our censors.

We imagine the problems of love are due to failure in a person's credentials. Not so. How many intellectual giants need the raw instinct of a so-called "dumb" wife or husband to sustain their very lives?

Our problem is to gain entrance to the higher reality of the heart and instinct where love flourishes endlessly. Pain, the pain of love points the way. This pain is unremitting in its demands. If we follow its direction, all of us can overcome most obstacles and join in a harmonious and joyful love relationship.

Love's Torments

How do we get beyond ego consciousness? How do we become *love itself* rather than loving?

In the springtime of romance, during early youth, we are carried away by our love. We are vulnerable to the core of our being. Later on, most people spend enormous energy trying to return to that same unqualified joy. Failure to regain that state may result in a lifetime of anger and depression. And we are quick to blame this depression on some deep-seated psychological problem in our personality or the personality of our mate.

To a degree this may be the case. But the basic difficulty is a good deal less complicated than we make it. We have replaced our intuitive response with mind response. In our effort to sustain love, we tend to depend on mind-motivated rather than instinct-motivated love.

All this is caused by anxiety. We fear that we will be abandoned by our lover or that we will lose our love-making capacity. To overcome this danger, we resort to mind engineered, possessive love. We justify all kinds of guilt creating political love, punitive love, exchange for services love, dependency love, cold love. All these may create excitement and intensity for a while, but they constrict and ultimately strangle love.

There was a time when love's torments were romanticized. Loss of a lover to another suitor or to family resistance was a lifetime tragedy. This is no longer the case. Today, we have no trouble *finding* lovers. But relationships are showing less and less duration.

Once again, our tendency is to misjudge the pain. The pain of love is entirely explicit in its directions. If we examine it carefully, it *does not* say, "discard your love, punish your love" or even "knock yourself out for love." It does say, "*enjoy* your love." This pain does not tell us to be false, to be over-solicitous, to be super brilliant, to be excessively amorous, to be bull headed in our love. It tells us very clearly to be *ourselves*. It tells us to enjoy the subtle feelings of our love exchange. It tells us *not to get wound up* in all kinds of premeditated approaches to love but to trust the moment *to itself*.

It is astonishing that love which is meant to provide elation and comfort provides such misery. It is even more astonishing that this misery is designed to *eliminate itself*, and we do not realize this. If both lovers will respond to the most serious oppression without theoretical jargon, without the insidious convictions that originate in thought, without the heated emotions that are aggravated by thought—if they leave it to their hearts and their feeling, the problem will right itself rapidly.

If there is a battle over a child's behavior, or over money, or even a career, or over who shall do such and such in the house, is this the time to win the battle at any cost? Or does the terrible pain that accompanies such a battle tell us that we are both betraying ourselves?

If we are both suffering from an overdose of possessive love, or duty love, or unfeeling love, or compulsive love, or depraved love, or manipulative love, isn't the inevitable pain asking us to back away from each other and let some living space enter the congested atmosphere? Surely it is not asking us to keep testing the *false* ties and to bind them even further.

If a man is frustrated by his job situation, must he take it out on his wife or run to another woman to restore his pride? Isn't the pain telling them that there is something meaningful and touching in the reverses that accompany all existence?

If a woman is no longer the beautiful sex kitten she was twenty years ago, is this the time for her to cause even greater pain by being vindictive with herself and her man? Or is her pain telling her to enjoy her new role as a mature woman or an old woman?

Finally, even if we are rejected and abandoned by our love, does the unbearable pain tell us to forever mull over our misfortune? Or is it imploring us to live out the kaleidoscope of our lives?

Love *must* include anger, argument, passion, hurt, puzzlement and even a bit of insanity. By all means! But our pain awareness can see humor in love's worst moments. It will not eliminate conflict, but it *can* put an end to panic, to repulsion and to ruin.

Our Misunderstood Sexuality

Unless sex is an involuntary, unmanipulated act, the sexual apparatus is undermined. One of the disasters of our society is the incessant battering which we suffer in the hands of psychologists, sexologists and pornographers. We are pelted with pronunciamentos from on high which declare with absolute certainty that:

a. Mechanically devised techniques can overcome frigidity, impotence, premature orgasm, sexual timidity and anything is all right as long as it provides orgasm.

b. Only sex that is rooted in love is workable.

a. Women must learn to accept one night stands, to surrender totally, to play every sexual game.

b. Women must quit being sexual objects.

a. Men are generally bestial, without real capacity for the subtleties of sex.

b. Men are highly sensitive creatures who have to be wooed.

a. Men progressively lose their sexuality after the age of eighteen. Women only reach sexual maturity in their late thirties.

b. Sexuality is constant.

And so it goes, ad infinitum. All these are intended to free us from sexual inhibitions. But they have intensified mind sex, the very thing they were supposed to overcome. This causes as much misery as puritanism. It is the core of our sexual malaise. Love has largely become a partnership of convenience, and sex a chore. "Get your rocks off, one way or another," we are told. The ineffable mystery of sex, the awareness of that overwhelming experience that perpetuates life itself is a *toilet function*!

Ultimately *instinct rebels* against this plastic sexuality. It *refuses* to participate because it has lost its *primary* role. If our minds become the driving force, if we put instinct in the back seat, instinct becomes more and more non-functioning. We suffer frigidity and impotence. Sex becomes a contest, a war, an area of cynicism; no longer an ecstatic article of faith, a spiritual anchor even for the atheist. We lose respect for the mysteries of our nature. We lose *our nature*.

Sex without premeditation, without guile, without devious cover-up is one of the primary gateways to reality. Freud and other psychologists insist that a tormented sexuality *must* cause neurosis. *Why* is this so? These scientists of the mind never defined *sexuality itself*.

The Eastern definition of sexuality, as explained by the Tantrics, is opposite to our own definition. We regard sex as a need, like hunger for food, which incidentally provides sense and ego gratification. But the Tantrics regard sex as a powerful, instinctual return to our ultimate reality, one of the highest forms of meditation. In fifteen minutes to an hour or more of uninterrupted coitus they seek a complete *loss* of ego. The object is to become so completely instinctual, so mindless that we merge with ultimate nature. This, they insist, is the definition of our sexuality, the return to *absolute essence, absolute oneness.*

Our love and sex tends to be frenetic. Many of us believe we have had a supreme experience when we join in punishing intercourse that moves rapidly to climax. We hardly know what it is to lie in coitus without any motion at all, waiting for our nature to *tell us*, utterly relaxed, utterly mindless. We have not discovered that the greatest sexual thrill of all is *no search* for thrills, that our unencumbered nature wants to take us to a fantastic realm where kicks and thrills are eclipsed by our indefinable *consciousness*, our oneness with the universe. Such sex is *always* infinitely satisfying. Such a love relationship lasts indefinitely. It is never jaded, never cynical. All the sexual difficulties, the sexual pains, are brilliantly demanding and direct the way to such love.

Sexual Difficulty

We think we know what we *want* from sex but we remain unsure. We feel we *must* have sexual release and yet we can't say precisely *why*. Somehow or other we achieve our frenzied orgasms but they are often followed by a faint, post-coital despondency, a gnawing yearning for something unrealized. If we suffer from reduced libido, frigidity, premature orgasm, impotence or a depraved relationship, we become seriously depressed or obsessive. We resort to weird outlets: superficial relationships, idiotic fantasy, compulsive masturbation, uncontrolled anger, overeating—all accompanied by mounting panic. Nothing agitates our body, mind and emotions more than this distress.

Is it *inevitable* that sexual love should be accompanied by difficulty? *Must* we grow tired of our mate? *Must* we withhold ourselves and indulge in negative games to sustain interest? *Must* each coitus be a production? *Must* there be sexual decline with age? Why this pain? What is it saying?

Does it point to some incompetence or does it point to distinct solutions?

Let us take some examples. If a man suffers from premature ejaculation, is he sexually lacking? Or does his over-eager anxiety create the problem? Does a woman who suffers from so-called frigidity face a similar anxiety? The problem then is *mental* anxiety, mental eagerness. But it isn't our self-conscious mind that is making love. It is the *entire autonomic system* including the primal or instinctive mind. The conscious mind is a subordinate factor. Is the pain of sexual frustration begging us to surrender our cortical function, to give up mind interference in favor of our reflexes, our instinct, our greater reality?

How? Will liquor do it? Drugs, will power, self analysis? To a degree, yes. But this could lead to major new problems. "Should I take one valium or two and will it be okay if I mix it with a martini?" "Will my black night gown turn him on or should I try my pale green chemise?" "Am I reacting to her with my child mind or with my adult mind?" And so on, ad infinitum. Thought interference is only being intensified.

If, instead, we *observe* our pain from moment to moment, does it tell us what we should do? Is it saying, "Please do less rather than more—better still, please do nothing." Or, "Stop being so damned loving—so damned solicitous—so damned charismatic!" Or is this pain invoking a question, "Who in blazes asked you to be so falsely masculine or so preciously feminine?"

If we do absolutely nothing except what is *ultimately comfortable*, what we are being *asked to do*, if we *do not* put ourselves out but simply function in such a way that there will *not be any pain signals*, our sexuality takes an extraordinary turn. All the ego-love-hate-problems of *making it* on a one to one basis evaporate. Instead of the burdens of mind sex or judgmental sex or raw determination sex, we discover the infinitely greater power of instinctive sex. Instead of functioning out of the doubtful strength of personal ego, we function out of the strength of universal ego. By responding fully to every pain injunction, the entire love relationship from the simplest exchange over breakfast orange juice to coitus that evening dramatically changes.

Yes it *is* possible for a man and woman to join in sexual intercourse that is virtually without any body movement (in a meditative state). Yes it is possible to move from this state to one in which there is no such thing as unilateral body movement. Whatever occurs proceeds in a precise harmony, driven by forces that rise from the inexplicable truth of one being. Such intercourse is devoid of all doubt, all questioning, all aggression, all timidity. It is beyond either pleasure or displeasure. It returns us to our first cause, that state where we want for nothing in the entire universe.

This is the furthest thing from duty love. As the Orientals put it, this is nature, Godhood. And once again the way is absolute and patient response to pain. This pain *insists* on mutuality of passion. It refuses to tolerate sexual cynicism (which is also cynicism of *our* entire existence) on the one hand, and refuses to tolerate over-sensitivity on the other hand. It will deliver and guarantee total tumescence from beginning to end with orgasm by both partners at any desired moment. Such instinctive sex is a godlike experience. It transcends all the difficulties of the day and all the likes and dislikes that are mind fabricated. Looks, clothes, perfume, wit, age, "sexiness" mean nothing. It is as absolute and overwhelming in its first experience as it is in every other experience. Ceaselessly our nature entreats us to engage in this open hearted supra-reality. And if we do not respond to this pain request, we inevitably suffer a beleaguered mind and a diminished soul.

In this sexual experience all must give way to the generative, genital, diencephalic, instinctive power of our cosmos. All the superficial mind games crumble before the majestic "I" principle - Function - Conscience - Kundalini. With infinitely subtle love that springs from our "world without end" we join in the stately dance of Being. We are our Omnipresent, Omnipotent reality. We are the Life-Fire, the *I am*—the *We are*!

Is this a mirage? Test it yourself. Put aside a weekend for meditative sleep and meditative sex. At least once each evening or once each morning allow no pain or tension to disturb your sexual experience. Let it guide you to ultimate, meditative, extended intercourse. Follow this with pain guided painless sleep and pain guided painless waking hours. It will do more for you than the two weeks of vacation for which you slave all year. Instead of a tense stomach, dry lips, aching muscles, an aching heart, dried-out sexuality and disillusionment towards the world, you will feel perfect physical, mental and emotional health, a sweeter-than-life vibe, a love and acceptance of life that will be nothing short of miraculous. There may be occasional lapses, but you will return to this again and again, year after year, time after time!

Chapter Eleven

ARTISTIC AND SPONTANEITY BLOCK

The pain of artistic block tells the artist that he or she is functioning without intuition. It demands a return to intuitive inspiration as the primary supply source. Every artist is forced to deal with this problem.

Because the creative artist is desperate to return to his or her professional function, there is a tendency to try to overcome the problem with intense self-analysis. But this causes an *even greater* excess of mind centered self-consciousness which is precisely what creates the problem in the first place. It *aggravates* the unproductive state.

What can we do now? A vacation, the stimulation of friends, a new love, a hilarious experience, love for a child, an intense sexual experience may work. It opens the heart, it releases constriction. But suppose the dreaded thing happens. *Nothing* works! Despair and non-productivity feed on each other. We have a severe case of artistic block.

This problem is not exclusive to artists. We are all endowed or spring from artistic genius, even if our medium is *not* one of the arts. Each of us has talents in which our natural grace functions with spontaneous perfection. We may be particularly good at being attractive or funny or being parents or friends. A waitress in an obscure roadside diner may perform her function with overwhelming charm and sensitivity. And down the road a hardware store may be run by a man whose knowledge and handling of his many products is utmost poetry. A thief, a scoundrel, a woebegone beggar, a panhandler, a prostitute, an alcoholic—they too! We all perform with absolute brilliance in *some area* of our daily lives. When we are truly spontaneous, each and every one of us is able to do a job, to utter a phrase, to execute a movement with mysterious perfection. We are all a collective genius—the collective life force. And when any one of us suffers a loss of spontaneity, we too suffer artistic block and its inevitable frustration.

What is the source of this misery? Is it that we are not thinking right or living right or doing right? Ultimately none of these. What we have lost, what our misery is crying for, is a return to a lost interrelatedness with the total stream of being. We have become unilateral—*me against the hostile world*. We are not plugged in to our universal miracle; the miracle in every human, every animal, every insect, every speck of dust. Our atmosphere has become too rarefied. Far better to "look homeward angel" as Thomas Wolfe put it, to return to plainness, to plain folk, to the unadorned drama of childhood, youth, adulthood and old age, to the millions of unheroic heroes, to the struggle for survival, yes, even to our most fundamental functions, chewing food, picking our teeth, belching, defecating, passing gas, sweating, breathing, copulating, sleeping, sneezing. We put down these functions, these instincts, but hidden there is the true miracle of our existence. And they include despair and hope, sickness and health, and the fear of dying.

It is not *me against the world*, it is *me the world*. Most of our misery is an anguished cry from our inner being to return to our essential nature. But the route for this return is difficult to find. The artist's stock in trade is uniqueness—to be one step apart. His misery is demanding that he return, at least for a time, to his ordinary being, to be as un-unique, as devoid of presumption, as anonymous as a lonely trucker driving into a strange town after several hundred miles on the road, grimy, discomforted, sick of his own thoughts, desperate for a toilet to relieve himself, any kind of cheap hamburger, and any human voice. He may be infinitely closer to our essential truth than a president delivering the State of the Union address, closer to feeling than our greatest playwrights.

How do we re-establish contact, how do we once more drink the milk of the realm? This gift of inspiration is an elusive Blue Bird. Chase it and it flies away. Ignore it and it lights on your shoulder singing its perfect song. All life derives from the sun and from mud. If we harness ourself to the sun alone, we will burn to a crisp. And mud alone will cause us to rot and decay. We lose our intuition when we are super special and we lose it when we are super cynical. The pain and misery of artistic block forces us to get deep into the mud and forces us to open our eyes to the sun—simultaneously.

There is no inspiration unless we join the mundane with the supra-mundane. Unless reality is as miraculous as the *supposedly* miraculous, we are frozen in ice. Unless we are as much *of* life as we are *in* life, our art is sterile. The miseries of artistic block *command* us, force us to exchange false idealism or cynicism for the magic in realism.

How?

This misery accomplishes its end by itself. It needs no help from us. It shoves us off the ledges of all our high places. It thrashes us within an inch of our lives. It brings our egos to point zero. If forces us to question every reference, every principle we ever held. Ultimately it forces us to discard *all* our principles. It floats every piece of mind garbage to the surface and for a period we can't tolerate ourselves. And finally, at absolute zero, absolute surrender, our life force takes over once more, and we are returned to *nadam*, to free flowing totality, to our pure being. In this state everything is okay, *right*! A rusting tin can fills us with radical awe as the sunlight catches it.

The yogis use surprisingly simple methods to expedite the process by which the sublime juice is flowing again. They make a frontal attack on the mind, on ego, on vanity, and the worst curse of all—spiritual vanity. Try going to a hard hitting Yoga or Buddhist retreat sometime. You rise at five-thirty AM, sit in silent meditation with fifty other people for an hour and a half, do some quite excruciating stretching exercise for another hour and a half, eat a modest breakfast (an apple and some cereal), work three hours at some totally menial task, chant for two hours like an absolute nobody, eat a modest dinner, listen to a twenty minute lecture and finally meditate another hour and a half before you stumble off to sleep.

After a week of this, your self-judgmental and world-judgmental ego will be pulverized. You will find glory in any other person's smile—or frown. You will sense a world you have long forgotten, unbelievably rich and intricate in every detail, breathlessly mysterious. You will appreciate the truth of suffering.

What has happened?

You have learned once again, and it takes constant relearning, that life rises out of life. You will have put an end to the game of self deception. You have acknowledged who you are, and who you *are not*. You are *now* coming from your totality, your status quo, from the common sense of your common sense; and you fully acknowledge pain and death and impermanence as a creative function.

Is there an alternative to a yoga-retreat, some other way to overcome artistic block?

Ultimately misery washes us all clean. It kills off our pretensions. It renders our ploys useless, reduces us to size, forces us to a new humility from which rises a new majesty. Yes, we *can* expedite the process. Try spending a day with "embarrassing" relatives, face their vulnerability; go to a simple church service and join the "gullible" people in their age-old ritual; share the doubtful pleasure of a summer walk on a boardwalk with "plain" people; give your attention to a "dumb" pet. You may wonder *who* is embarrassing, gullible, plain and dumb. You may rediscover *that common clay* from which all rises. You may rediscover your collective being and be inspired again.

Chapter Twelve

FAITH HEALING, TRANQUILIZERS, BIO-FEEDBACK, RECREATION

Faith healing, Christian Science, recreation, laying on of hands, tranquilizers, mind expanding drugs, bio-feedback and pain awareness have a common function. All these release the autonomic system from the machinations of the mind. They are a means by which we achieve *involuntary* function.

Christian Science and faith healing do not necessarily induce a special dispensation from God, a reward for prayer and obeisance. Prayer and faith are another means by which we are released from psychosomatic constriction. When we invest intense faith in an outside force, we have partially relinquished ourselves to our *instinctive force*. (Unless the faith is an ego trip.) If there is sufficient intensity, the constriction gives way to cure.

If we believe that equilibrium and God or Godhood are identical, this is a spiritual process. Intense worship of Christ, for example, brings a devout Christian to a high level of surrender. In place of self-doubt, self-hate, and self-consciousness, there is the purest Christ Consciousness, a flow of life force. Whether we label this pure flow a simple psychosomatic cure, Tao, Samadhi, Satori, Christ Consciousness, or God does not matter. I find supreme hypocrisy in the smug healer who mocks the success of other religious, medical or psychological disciplines when he knows full well that there is a common force that makes all these techniques possible. With practise, anybody can feel the flow of the life force current, and can judge whether it is free flowing or obstructed.

Hopefully we are entering an era in which healing will not be the exclusive moneymaking business it has been, when we will show primary respect for the miraculous physio-pyscho-spiritual nature which is our common reality. If the same illness responds to faith healing, to a tranquilizer, to psychiatry, to bio-feedback, to a vacation in the Bahamas, and to pain awareness with equal effectiveness, then all power to all six methods. The method worked! Who is to say that the cure—let us say the release of a muscle spasm in the neck—was not absolutely identical in every case, though the methods appear to be so irreconcilably varied.

Bio-feedback measures our various tensions: muscle tension, increased heartbeat, skin vessel constriction, eyeball dilation, etc. It allows us to observe what our body is doing (telling us) with the assistance of dials and buzzers that signal our eyes and ears that something is not normal. Bio-feedback has been used with varying success in the treatment of high blood pressure, headaches, stress, muscle contraction and other difficulties.

In a very distinct sense bio-feedback can be linked to pain scanning. Much of what the bio-feedback machines tell us can be *sensed* if we are aware of our pain signals. The two techniques complement each other. Bio-feedback is useless if its instruction doesn't become habit. We cannot carry these machines wherever we go. Pain awareness is the process that carries out the lessons of the bio-feedback experience. Conversely, the bio-feedback machine may help reveal a neglected area of pain awareness.

Bio-feedback has certain limitations—as do each of the techniques we are discussing. It is a measurement of *raw energy*. It does not measure feeling. The energy of one pain tension may be equal to another, but the quality of the pain, the subtleties of tone cannot be measured by the instruments.

Our minds cannot translate the infinite complexities of our actions, desires, disappointments, frustrations, joys, etc. But our *feeling* has this capacity. It is infinitely more brilliant than mind or machine. For example, bio-feedback machines are able to record alpha wave phenomena but they cannot begin to record the infinitely subtle perceptions which the alpha wave imparts.

Chapter Thirteen

THE MALAISE AND THE RAGE OF MODERN SOCIETY

With all our material progress, discontent is rampant throughout the world. Children are discontented with their parents, parents with their children, people with work and women with housework. There is sexual war, a contempt for love and tenderness. There is lifelessness and because of this there is an undertow of tremendous rage.

If we refuse to enter into relationships and to suffer the pain of these relationships—if we keep our cool, suffer no emotional penetration from others, make no bonds, avoid allegiances, barricade ourselves with drugs, substitute pizzas, TV and other ersatz sensation for our reality—where will we be? Miserable! Static! Hostile! Suicidal! Bitterly depressed! Precisely where we are today!

Why?

Because we cannot function apart from the mainspring of our being, apart from that joy and pain by which our instinct, our essential form, or if you will, our Godhood functions. Because we cannot substitute sensation for feeling, intelligence for feeling, poise for feeling, religious vanity for feeling. Because love and the pain of love, hope and the pain of hope, generosity and the pain of generosity, openness and the pain of openness—all these are the mysterious thing that we *are*! Because we are truncated unless we are in touch with our actuality. *Because we—our nature is the soul of the universe.*

A piece of stone is unperturbed, uncommitted. But we are not stone. We cannot build a pain-proof society. Underneath the world's blasé exterior there is black depression and hostility. This black pain is screaming at us to be whole hearted, to make mistakes, to get hooked again and again with commitments, to make some act of faith to the mysterious cosmos. We are all overcome by life sooner or later, reduced, yes battered. The secret is to *be battered*, to give up being defensive, and to be intoxicated by the reality in our reality.

The pain of defensive action is telling us to amputate all our survival ploys, to throw ourselves to the wind, to be whatever *is*! Our world malaise tells us every day that there is nothing to hold on to, absolutely nothing! We are all part of a perpetual motion force. We *are* that force. We can't stop the train or jump off the train. *We are the Train*! If we make the slightest attempt to halt the train we suffer pain. How can we stop our own momentum?

Even if the world will be blown to bits by atom bombs tomorrow, our perpetual motion will still remain intact. Even if not one blade of grass remains, the time must come when out of the neutrons and atoms some cockroach looking creature will once again say, "What a fantastic train, oh what a train!"

Chapter Fourteen

SUMMARY

Pain awareness will work with amazing effectiveness if the following axioms are observed:

1. Pain is a guide not an enemy.

2. The pain *tells you*, you do not tell the pain.

3. Theorizing about pain will distort your response to pain.

4. Fear of pain, fighting pain, anger at pain, ignoring or masking pain will distort your response to pain.

5. You cannot be impatient with pain. You must allow whatever time is required to permit it to perform its function.

6. The method by which we respond to pain is simply to feel it deeply and to respond to those feelings. Pain is self-eliminating.

7. Pain is a feeling. Feelings derive directly from diencephalic and autonomic function. Autonomic function contains the wisdom of billions of years of evolution. Vedantic teaching

claims that this autonomic evolutionary function—this natural law—is identical to our total reality, or for those who prefer, to our Total Reality.

8. Unless we concede our being to God or Godhead or nature, or Christ or Buddha or instinct, or this total reality, we cannot perceive this process.

The function and the success of pain awareness could not be more direct and more obvious. Unfortunately our manipulating mind obscures the process. A hundred times or more, each and every hour, we react to our body or to our emotional need. We scratch ourselves, or relieve a cramped foot, or make an overdue telephone call, or quench our thirst, or sit back and relax, or open our hearts to a loved one. This is the *very act of living.* This is our make-up.

Those who feel that response to instinct is a permissive concept do not realize that *nature itself* is ruthless in its disciplines. We may feel we are escaping nature's narrow line, but every step away from this line automatically creates a greater pull to the opposite direction. We are punished *by* our sin, not for our sin. If we eat too much, we get a stomach ache. The process of instinctive nature cannot be violated. The laws of our omni-psychology are as strict as the laws of our omni-science.

Chapter Fifteen

CONCLUSION

These are enormously exciting times. All of us can walk the world with a new awe—as great as the wonder felt by the Biblical Patriarchs. The revealed mysteries of science indicate vast numbers of interrelated energy planes moving at lightning speed. Also revealed within the inner being of each and every one of us are instinctive planes that are central to this universe. The realities of the outer world and the realities of our inner world are not separated by any boundary. We and science and the unknown are inseparable. We live at the dawn of the age of supramentality. All this is even more exciting than the dawn of scientific discovery.

Our new world promises to be an enormously pragmatic world. It will not live in dreams or high-flown phrases or holy exhortations. It will find this world perfect as it is, marvelously exciting in its seeming imperfection. Physics and metaphysics will be merged. We will have a *cosmic understanding* that will answer the enigma of our existence and we will find hilarious delight in our predicament. We will revel in our enigmas even as we are being tortured by them.

On that day, we will find no need to reach out for answers of any kind. We will stand four-square in our instinctive being which itself is absolute reality. Reality does not have to be explained to reality. The function of a kite does not have to be explained to the kite. The function of our being does not have to be explained to our being. There is nothing fancy or remote about the supreme reality. It is supreme because it is reality—the *only* reality—*our very reality*. What else can possibly be supreme? The primitives who actually lived with their deep feelings before the advent of witch doctors may have been a hundred times more in touch with their being-reality than we are. To give up the apple of the tree of knowledge, is to gain *all knowledge*.

It is only instinct that can lead us to Instinct. And it is only our intimations—pain, pleasure, feelings—that can lead us to instinct.

Either there are no problems at all, or all existence is an insoluble problem because it is an inevitable march to oblivion. This should cause *incessant pain*! The sweeter life is, the more infuriated we should become. But we *do not* suffer incessant pain. We *do* accept and even laugh at our outrageous predicament more than we realize. Doesn't the pain somehow resolve our problem, even as it seems to cause the problem? Doesn't it *force* us to see the game in our game? Doesn't it mysteriously explain our inevitabilities? Doesn't it tell us to quit being martyrs, to "get off it." The loss of pain's function, the loss of our feelings' purpose, is the mistake of contemporary mankind. The animal and plant kingdom never gave this up and they survive with dignity, without self-hate. Mankind suffers mass hysteria. Mankind is suicidal.

We are not loving, we are love itself. We are not sexy, we are sex itself. We do not suffer painful or pleasurable experience, we are pain and pleasure itself. We are not dying, we are death itself. The function of our moment and the collective moment are identical. We can trust the world to the world, we can trust the universe to the universe, and we can trust ourselves to ourselves. We wouldn't want one thing any other way than it is because it is *our* scene, *our* dance, *our* orgy party, *our* undending bash! And, as the pain will teach us, it is our divinity!

The day is coming when we will read our feelings with much more perception than we read our crazy cat, reference laden, information collecting and information confusing mind. On that day we will not fear our feelings. They tell us of our infinite worlds. *Ours*, we create them all! On that day we will quit throwing away our miraculous instinctive capacity to voices other than our own voice. On that day we will cherish the entire pain-pleasure, moral-immoral, good-bad, right-wrong, life-death, being-non-being, creator-created, designer-designed opposites of our individual-collective being. On that day we will be free of limitations and afflictions. We will all share the amazing logic of pain and the ineffable logic of nature.

The road back to our instinctive Eden will be filled with obstacles. At every turn we will find our intimate friend the snake (ego, intellect) sitting with another shiny jelly apple: assorted pain killers, cars, pizza pies, uppers-downers, violent films, a new psychological theory, Caribbean vacation—ten thousand panaceas! Yes, all these are fine, provided we do not lose sight of the majestic reality that supports the entire foundering ship of fools, provided we view all panaceas with humor, provided we utilize them to enhance rather than to detract from our instinctive experience. Provided we periodically realize we *never* lost our Eden.

Anti Finem

There is a tendency by yogic and other cosmological writers to freely make broad assumptions. I plead guilty to having done just this. I have no defense. If I had had the time and the training to eliminate all the one-sided statements and to qualify all the partially provable premises in this book, I would feel much better at this moment. For this I apologize to all who labor so diligently with the razor sharp complexities of their disciplines.

But civilization is shortchanging itself by replacing respect for the unknown with worship of ten thousand disjointed technologies. We are disregarding the unifying element that makes all these technologies possible. Hypothesis has become an almost forgotten art that desperately needs reviving if we are to deal more effectively with daily existence—if we are to live more hopeful lives.